St

Manage

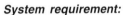

System requirement:
- **Windows XP or above**
- **Power DVD player (Software)**
- **Windows Media Player 10.0 version or above**
- **Quick time player version 6.5 or above**

Accompanying CD ROM is playable only in Computer and not in CD player.

Kindly wait for few seconds for CD to autorun. If it does not autorun then please do the following:
- Click on my computer
- Click the **drive labelled JAYPEE** and after opening the drive, kindly double click the file **Jaypee**

Step by Step®

Management of Burns

Sujata Sarabahi
MBBS MS MCh DNB MNAMS
Plastic Surgeon
Department of Burns and Plastic Surgery
Safdarjung Hospital, New Delhi, India

SP Bajaj
MBBS MS MCh FRCS (Glas)
Ex-Professor and Head
Department of Burns and Plastic Surgery
Safdarjung Hospital, New Delhi, India
Ex-President, National Association of Burns India (2000-2001)

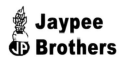

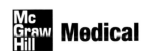

© 2009, Jaypee Brothers Medical Publishers
First published in India in 2009 by

Jaypee Brothers Medical Publishers (P) Ltd.

Corporate Office
4838/24 Ansari Road, Daryaganj, **New Delhi** - 110002, India, +91-11-43574357

Registered Office
B-3 EMCA House, 23/23B Ansari Road, Daryaganj, **New Delhi** 110 002, India
Phones: +91-11-23272143, +91-11-23272703, +91-11-23282021,
+91-11-23245672, Rel: +91-11-32558559 Fax: +91-11-23276490, +91-11-23245683
e-mail: jaypee@jaypeebrothers.com, Visit our website: www.jaypeebrothers.com

First published in USA by The McGraw-Hill Companies, 2 Penn Plaza, New York, NY 10121.
Exclusively worldwide distributor except South Asia (India, Nepal, Sri Lanka, Bhutan, Pakistan, Bangladesh, Malaysia).

ISBN-13: 978-0-07-163430-4
ISBN-10: 0-07-163430-4

Dedicated to
All the patients who
have been treated by us

Preface

Man's ability to ignite fire was probably his first step towards civilization. Fire helped nomadic man to settle down, preserve, hold and cook his food. However, during the process of close proximity with fire, the energy source, man kept injuring himself from fire and sustaining burns. Today's incidence of burns and how we manage burns is an indirect indication of how a society's health care policy takes care of its people.

Burn destroys not only the skin and other structures but it leaves behind permanent scar of injury which not only hampers the patient physically but also breaks them mentally and emotionally. The trauma and pain suffered by all the patients who have been treated by us has inspired us to write this book so that every medical practitioner is able to manage burns in the initial stages.

In this book we are providing step by step understanding about burns, how it affects the human body, how to manage and rehabilitate a burn victim. This book provides practical and workable solutions which are deliberately kept simple and at some places complex situations have been over-simplified so that it becomes user-friendly and the basic management of burns can be accomplished not only by Plastic Surgeons but also by General Surgeons and General Physicians.

Wherever there are controversies, different views have been given but emphatically one view is provided which we feel is better. We have avoided dogmas and our aim has been to provide simplified methods in developing scientific temper for management of burns not only by Plastic Surgeons but also by General Surgeons and General Practitioners as well.

We are thankful to Dr RP Narayan and Dr VK Tiwari for their constant support and encouragement.

Sujata Sarabahi
SP Bajaj

Contents

CHAPTER 1

Introduction to Burns

DEFINITION

Burns is any injury to skin by an energy source. This source of energy could be:

A. Heat —which could be by fire or by hot liquids
B. Chemicals
C. Electricity
D. Lasers
E. Friction
F. Radiation.

CLASSIFICATION

Depending on the type of energy the burns can be classified into:

A. Thermal burns –by dry heat, fire, lasers and steam
B. Scalds –by hot liquids
C. Electrical burns—by low or high voltage burns
D. Chemical burns – by acids, alkali or ionic compounds
E. Radiation burns
F. Friction burns.

Burns may involve the different layers of skin and has varied effects on the skin and may be the deeper structures. The amount of damage will be directly proportional to the amount of energy released by the energy source which will depend upon the temperature of the source and the duration of contact. The higher the temperature, greater is the degree and depth of damage. Also, longer the duration of contact with the source, the more severe the damage.

Considering the anatomy of skin (Fig. 1.1), it can be simply said to have two main layers, i.e. epidermis and

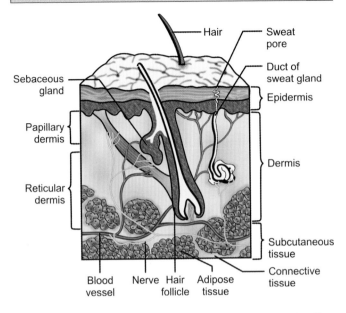

Fig. 1.1: Anatomy of normal skin showing epidermal papillae, superficial papillary dermis and deep reticular dermis. Sweat glands, sebaceous glands and hair follicles penetrate the dermis and subcutaneous fat to varying depth

dermis. Epidermis is made of dead cornified cells and a basal layer of rapidly dividing live columnar cells. The dermis consists of collagen, elastic fibers, nerve endings and blood vessels. The epidermis invaginates into the dermis to a certain extent in the form of rete ridges and thus divides it into a superficial layer called papillary dermis and deeper layer called reticular dermis. The epithelial appendages invaginating into the dermis include hair follicles, sweat glands and sebaceous glands.

Though the epidermis and dermis are intimately related, they come from two different stocks embryologically and work and function quite differently. Epidermis is protective and closes the wound. Dermis on the other hand is supportive and provides strength to the skin. Epidermis has the power of regeneration when damaged and hence leaves no tell tale story of damage, whereas dermis has no power of regeneration.

The proportion of epidermis and dermis is different in different parts of the body and even in the dermis, the proportion of papillary and reticular dermis is different in different parts of the body. More the element of epithelial cells, quicker is the healing process, e.g. burns of face heal very quickly because of greater availability of epithelial cells.

Burns have been broadly classified all over the world by different authors according to the level of damage in the skin layers into:

A. *First degree burns* (Figs 1.2A and B) which are also called *epidermal burns.* These are limited only to the most superficial layers of epidermis and heal spontaneously within 7 days because of abundance of epithelial cells which regenerate very fast. So this healing is by regeneration only and does not leave any scars.

B. *Second degree burns* (Figs 1.3A to 1.4B) which involve epidermis and varying depths of dermis. These have been further divided into superficial and deep second degree burns.

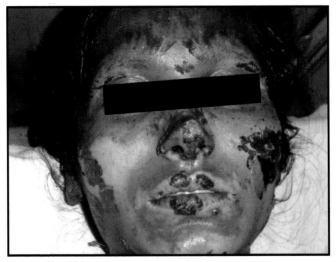

Fig. 1.2A: Epidermal or first degree burn of face, healed in 5 days without any scars

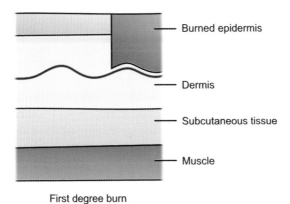

First degree burn

Fig. 1.2B: Anatomical representation of first degree burns involving only epidermis

C. *Third degree burns* (Figs 1.6A and B) involving entire epidermis and dermis and all dermal appendages so there is no spontaneous healing of the wound, leaving an ulcer. Since the entire thickness of skin is burned with no tissue left for repair and regeneration, these will require skin grafting or will close by contractures wherein two raw surfaces fuse together.

D. *Fourth degree burns* (Figs 1.7A and B) damage extends beyond the skin till muscle, fascia or bone. However, this is not a universally accepted term and is not used.

Here we have preferred to simplify the classification of burns into two basic types:

A. Burns which heal on their own and do not require any surgical intervention are *Superficial burns.*

B. Burns which do not heal on their own and require some sort of surgical intervention are *Deep burns.*

Superficial burns are again divided into two types:

i. *Superficial dermal or superficial partial thickness burns (Figs 1.3A to D)* which involve the epidermis and the papillary dermis. These also heal on their own by epithelial growth from the abundant skin appendages but slower than epidermal burns because as we go deeper the number of epithelial cells decreases and amount of connective tissue increases. Therefore the healing in these burns is by regeneration and repair both of which gives a scar. These usually heal in 14 days.

ii. *Deep dermal or deep partial thickness burns (Figs 1.4A and B)* which involve the epidermis and papillary dermis and reticular layer of dermis to varying depths. A few sweat glands and hair follicles are left behind

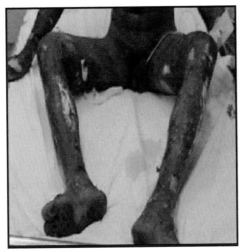

Fig. 1.3A: Superficial second degree or superficial partial thickness burns of lower limbs

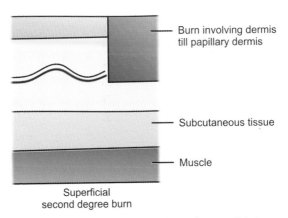

— Burn involving dermis till papillary dermis

— Subcutaneous tissue

— Muscle

Superficial
second degree burn

Fig. 1.3B: Anatomical representation of superficial second degree burns involving epidermis and superficial or papillary dermis

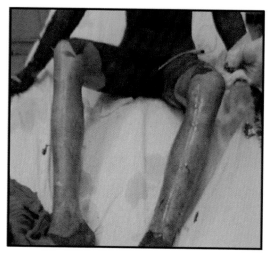

Fig. 1.3C: Same patient after debridement of loose dead epidermis giving a shiny, pink appearance

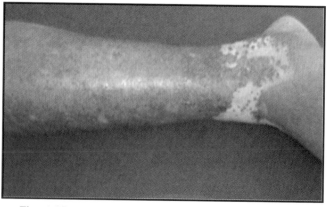

Fig. 1.3D: Healed wounds after 14 days in the same patient showing well settled scars

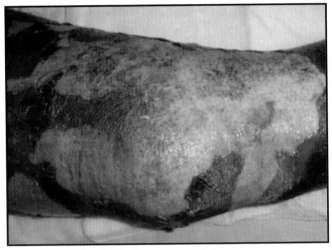

Fig. 1.4A: Deep second degree or deep partial thickness burns

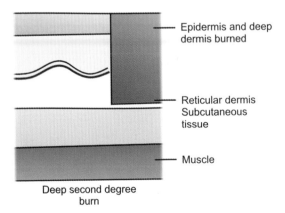

Epidermis and deep dermis burned

Reticular dermis
Subcutaneous tissue

Muscle

Deep second degree burn

Fig. 1.4B: Anatomical representation of deep second degree burns involving epidermis, superficial dermis and deep dermis to varying depths

in the reticular dermis from which there is marginal spread of epithelium which gradually covers the wound. This process usually takes more than 6 weeks and the healing takes place by extensive repair which lead to hypertrophic scarring (Fig. 1.5).

ASSESSMENT OF BURN DEPTH

Techniques for Assessing Burn Depth

There are many methods for assessing depth of burns but none of them are used as they are all experimental techniques. These include:

Laser Doppler, thermography and fluorescein fluorometry which uses the principle of amount of blood flow to assess the depth of damage in the skin. Ultrasound and dye studies have been used in animals and do not give a precise idea regarding depth of burn. Histological

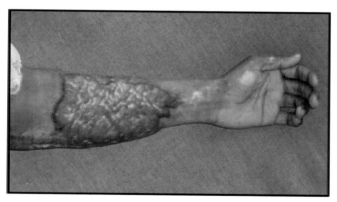

Fig. 1.5: Areas of deep second degree burns healed with hypertrophic scarring

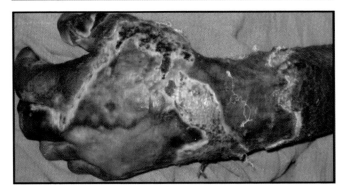

Fig. 1.6A: Third degree or full thickness burns of hand

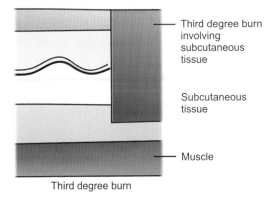

Third degree burn involving subcutaneous tissue

Subcutaneous tissue

Muscle

Third degree burn

Fig. 1.6B: Anatomical representation of third degree burns involving all layers of skin and varying depth of subcutaneous tissue

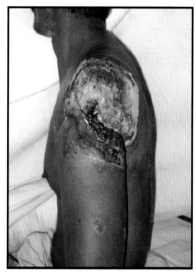

Fig. 1.7A: Fourth degree burns involving skin as well as underlying muscle and bone

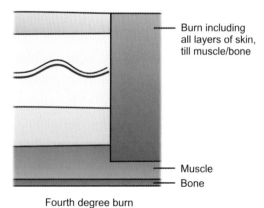

Burn including all layers of skin, till muscle/bone

Muscle

Bone

Fourth degree burn

Fig. 1.7B: Anatomical representation of fourth degree burns

wound biopsy seems to be the best diagnostic tool but is not practical to use in clinical practise. All these methods are good supportive tools to decide about depth but clinical evaluation remains the most accurate method of assessing depth of burn.

History: Includes the material causing the injury, temperature of the agent as well as the duration of contact. The depth of burns is directly proportional to both these factors. A prolong contact with low heat may cause deeper burns while an ultrashort contact with intense heat may lead to only superficial burns. The latent heat of a liquid agent causing the injury is an important factor as the more the latent heat, the more is the depth of damage, e.g. the latent heat of boiling oil and hot coffee is more than that of boiling water, so hot oil and hot coffee causes deeper burns compared to hot water. Partial thickness burns are typically caused by fire, scalds and brief exposure to flame or radiant heat. Full thickness burns are caused by prolonged exposure to heat, intense radiation, electric burns or immersion scalds.

Age is also an important factor as agents which cause superficial burns in adults may cause deep burns in children and elderly because of thinness of skin in children and atrophy of epithelial and dermal elements in the elderly.

Signs and symptoms: Vary according to the degree of burns.

Epidermal burns are characterized by erythema and severe local pain. Commonest example is sunburn. These heal in 7 days (Fig. 1.8).

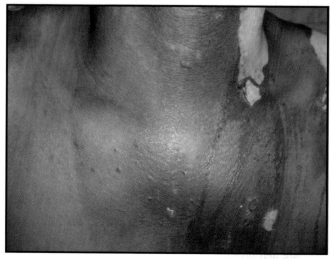

Fig. 1.8: Sunburn (epidermal burn) of neck with hyperemia and burning pain

Superficial partial thickness burns are also very painful because of exposed nerve endings and are very sensitive to temperature changes and touch. They are characterized by erythema with blister formation and when these are removed the epidermis below is weeping, glistening, bright red or pink. These areas appear edematous and raised above the normal surrounding skin. Majority of the hair cannot be pulled out because most of the hair follicles are embedded deep in the reticular dermis, which is not effected in this injury. These burns are very sensitive to pinprick (pinprick test of Douglas Jackson) (Fig. 1.9).

Deep partial thickness burn wounds are comparatively difficult to diagnose. Though typically waxy white, they

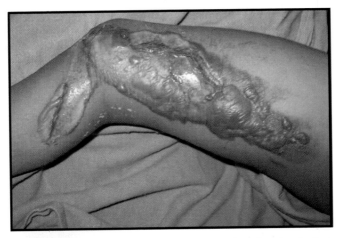

Fig. 1.9: Superficial dermal burns of lower leg showing typical blisters and underlying glistening red surface which blanches on pressure. These heal within two weeks

may be reddish with no capillary blanching and sometimes salt and pepper look. The areas are soft and elastic in consistency. They are sensitive to pressure but insensitive to touch and pain because of destruction of nerve endings. Most of the hair can be pulled out easily (Figs 1.10 and 1.11).

Full thickness burn wounds are hard and dry, brown colored or deep red, parchment like and transluscent with visible thrombosed dermal vessels. The eschar is inelastic and appears depressed below the normal skin and may compress on the deeper tissues when edema forms beneath it. These burns are also anesthetic to touch and pinprick (Figs 1.12 and 1.13).

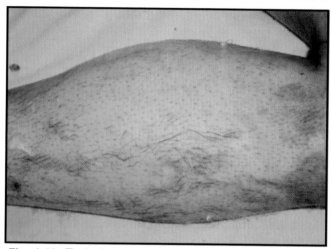

Fig. 1.10: Typical deep dermal burns of leg with dry waxy white appearance with no blistering and loose hair

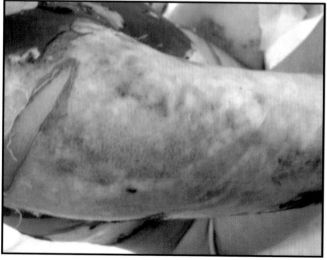

Fig. 1.11: Deep dermal burns of upper limb

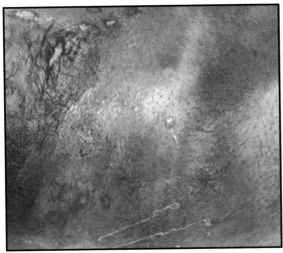

Fig. 1.12: Deep or full thickness burns showing hard, dry parchment like surface with visible thrombosed vessels

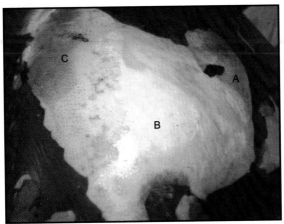

Fig. 1.13: Mixed superficial and deep burns of the back. (A) superficial dermal, (B) deep dermal and (C) full thickness burns

The deep partial thickness burn wounds can get converted into full thickness wounds by exposure to dry air or by infection. Therefore they have to be kept moist at all times and protected from contamination by microorganisms.

Reburn or Burn in Grafted Areas or Donor Areas (Fig. 1.14): Are usually deeper than the burns on other areas of the body because the thickness of skin is already reduced. It is mainly the epidermis and dermal appendages which are less because of previous burn and therefore a second degree burn is more likely to be deeper and the healing takes longer than usual and with further bad scars, either hypertrophic or keloids.

Laser burns (Fig. 1.15): Burns caused by lasers are basically thermal burns where laser energy is used for other purposes like hair removal or resurfacing or vascular or

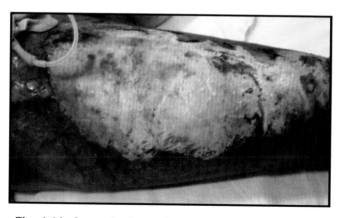

Fig. 1.14: Case of reburn of thigh already scarred due to previous burns. These take a longer time to heal

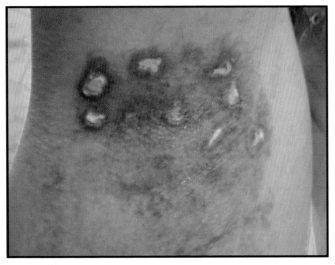

Fig. 1.15: Laser burns in axilla during hair removal. Multiple areas of deep burns which take a long time to heal. Can be managed with conservative management alone

pigmented lesions and heat released is dissipated into the normal skin leading to skin burns. The damage to the skin will depend upon the energy released by the laser, therefore these can be superficial burns which are more common or deep dermal when the energy used is very high, which take a long time to heal. Therefore wet gauze should be kept in surrounding skin thus isolating the treatment field as in resurfacing and treating pigmented or vascular lesions. In case of hair removal cold air blast is to be given along with the laser beam to nullify the effects of heat.

Fires also have been reported with use of lasers whenever there are flammable substances present in the operating field like oxygen used during anesthesia, dry gauze, alcohol, perfume, nail polish. Hence fire extinguishers should always be available near by.

Assessment of Body Surface Area Burned

Burns is a three-dimensional injury. There is a transverse and vertical dimension which can be described in terms of body surface area. The third dimension is the depth of burns, i.e first, second and third degree burns. The importance lies in the fact that the superficial burns heal on their own and deep burns require surgical intervention.

The extent of body surface area (BSA) burns can be estimated in different ways but the simplest and most universal technique which can be used by any individual is by the palmar aspect of the patients hand (with fingers closed) which forms 1 percent of his or her BSA (Fig. 1.17).

The next most common technique is the Wallace's "*Rule of 9*" (Fig. 1.16). This divides the body surface into eleven equal areas each of which is 9 percent of the total or in multiples of 9, e.g. each upper limb is 9 percent of the TBSA, each thigh is 9 percent of TBSA, each lower leg is 9 percent of TBSA, head and neck is 9 percent, front of chest is 9 percent, back of chest is 9 percent, front of abdomen is 9 percent and back of trunk is 9 percent. The perineal area is remaining 1 percent of TBSA.

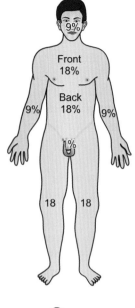

Fig. 1.16: Line diagram showing 'Rule of 9 '. Whole body is divided into eleven areas each of 9 percent and perineum is 1 percent

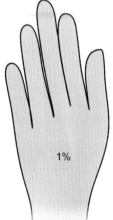

Fig. 1.17: Palmar aspect of hand with fingers closed depicting 1percent of TBSA (total burn surface area)

However, this technique cannot be applied for children because of the proportionately larger surface area of head and neck and smaller area of limbs. Hence, modification is done for calculating BSA burned in children. In an infant the head and neck is 19 percent of TBSA and lower limb is 10 percent of TBSA. The simplest method for calculation is to subtract 1 percent from head and neck and adding 1 percent to lower limb for every year after 1 year of age. This has been used in the *Lund and Browder* charting technique. *Rule of 5* (Figs 1.18A and B) has also been used though infrequently. According to this rule, the body is divided into 20 areas of 5 percent each by dividing the body into coronal and sagittal planes.

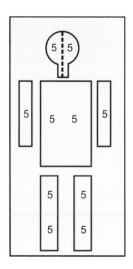

Fig. 1.18A: Line diagram of a child showing 'Rule of 5' in anterior view. Body is divided into 20 areas of 5 percent each

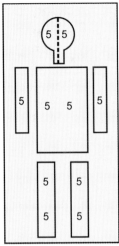

Fig. 1.18B: Line diagram of a child showing 'Rule of 5' in posterior view. Body is divided into 20 areas of 5 percent each

Another situation in which calculating the burned area can be a problem is in an amputee in whom the above formulas will give a deceptively higher percentage of burned area. In a normal patient as per 'Rule of 9' the total body is divided into 11 areas of 9 percent each, giving a total of 11 × 9 + 1 percent of perineal area = 100 percent BSA. In an amputee, according to the amount of limb loss the total BSA is reduced, e.g. if one lower limb is lost, surface left will be approx. 10 × 9 = 90 percent. So percentage of surface burnt will be calculated accordingly out of 90. If only face is burnt in an individual with one upper limb amputated, then percentage burns will be:

Out of 100 —— area burnt is 9

Therefore out of 90 —— area burnt = 9 × 90/100 = 8.1 percent

Zones of Damage (Jackson) (Fig. 1.19)

These vary due to the difference in heat transfer. In any damage due to heat, first there is hyperemia followed by stasis and then coagulation of tissue. Since the greatest heat transfer is in the centre there is irreversible cell death leading to *Zone of coagulation* in the middle. This is surrounded by an area of increased inflammatory reaction called *Zone of stasis*. This is further surrounded by an area of minimal cell involvement with early spontaneous recovery and is called *Zone of hyperemia*. If wound gets infected or is exposed to dry air, the zone of stasis can get converted to area of complete cell death.

Assessment of Severity of Burns (Table 1.1)

The severity of burn injury is determined by many factors. The most important being the quantum of tissue burnt in which the body surface area burnt gives the best

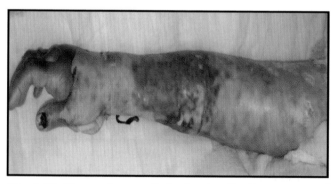

Fig. 1.19: Burns of upper limb showing the three zones of damage —central zone of coagulation, surrounded by zone of stasis and peripheral zone of hyperemia

Table 1.1: Criteria for severity of burns

Major	Moderate	Minor
• Partial thickness burns >25% BSA in adults	• Partial thickness burns 15-25% BSA in adults	• Partial thickness burns <15% in adults
• Partial thickness burns >15-20% BSA in children and elderly	• Partal thickness burns of 10-15% BSA in children and elderly	• <10% BSA in children and elderly
• Full thickness burns >10% BSA	• Full thickness burns of 2-10% BSA	• Full thickness burns <2% BSA
• High voltage electric burns	• Associated medical problems predisposing patient to infection	
• Inhalational injury		
• Burns of face, eyes, ears, hands, perineum and feet		
• Associated major soft tissue injury		
• Associated chest, abdominal and skeletal trauma		
• Circumferential burns of limbs, neck and chest		
• Patient to be referred to burn center for further management	• Hospital admission required	• OPD management

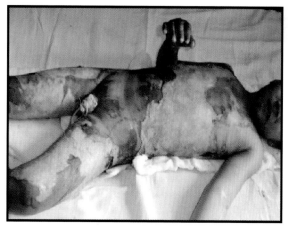

Fig. 1.20: Extensive burns in a child requiring admission

assessment, severity being directly proportional to BSA. However, depth is also very important. The deeper the burns, the worse the prognosis and may even lead to amputation of a body part. Severity is also related to age of the patient. In elderly and children, burns behave differently from that in adults. The elderly can succumb to even small burns because of other associated medical ailments. In infants and children, even though healing may be quick with a better ability to respond to trauma, however, because of poor ratio of BSA to blood volume they may succumb more quickly to initial shock phase (Fig. 1.20).

CHAPTER 2

Physiological Changes following Burns

There are basically two effects following burns:
1. Local response
2. General response

Following burns there is a sudden increase in body temperature which causes vasodilatation to dissipate heat. Further rise in temperature may start inflammatory reaction. The events take place in the following manner:

- Local edema formation starts within 1-3 hours due to:
  — Vasodilatation
  — Increased vascular permeability
  — Increased microvascular activity
- No reflow phenomenon occurring between 12-24 hours causing local tissue ischemia which may lead to necrosis.
- Platelets removed from circulation then lead to hemostasis and local thrombosis. This is a period of transformation which may lead to adhesions on endothelial cells, platelets and leukocytes.
- The late phase includes wound repair which has a high rate of wound perfusion.

Extracellular Changes (Flow chart 2.1)

Factors which increase capillary permeability are:
- Direct thermal damage
- Histamine and serotonin released from mast cells, platelets, gut and brain
- Plasma proteases and polypeptides
- Prostaglandin E.

The increase in capillary permeability following thermal burns is limited mainly to the burned area in case of <30

Flow chart 2.1: Showing physiological response to burns

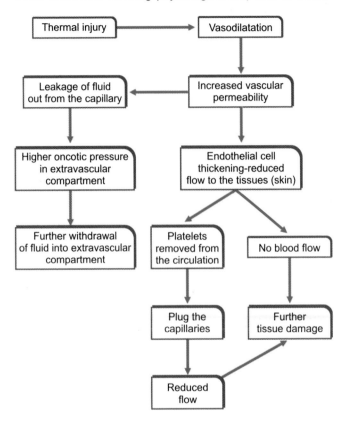

percent burns but is generalized all over the body in case burns is > 30 percent TBSA although the greatest change is seen in the injured skin itself. The loss of the capillary integrity causes proteins /colloidal substances of more than 150,000 molecular weight to escape into extravascular space. There is also loss of fluid from intravascular compartment to the extravascular compartment causing rapid accumulation of edema fluid in subcutaneous tissue deep to the burned surface. It has also been hypothesized that the increase in burn tissue osmotic pressure due to sodium binding to injured collagen also causes rapid fluid loss. The fluid and protein losses are greatest in the first 6-8 hours because of increase vascular permeability and increased interstitial osmotic pressure. These changes in capillary permeability start returning towards normal by 48 hrs and within 72 hours it is completely back to normal.

Because of leakage of plasma proteins into extra-vascular space, the colloid oncotic pressure in the extra-vascular space increases whereas intravascular colloid oncotic pressure decreases. The translocation of fluid causes edema in non-burned skin all over the body as well. The intravascular volume can therefore be expanded by transfusing like fluids, i.e plasma or colloids.

Intracellular Changes

In burns different type of cells are damaged because of change in the transmembrane potential of the cells following burns. There is a disturbance in the sodium-potassium ATP ase pump in the cells of the burned tissue as well as in cells of distant site from the burned surface. The normal transmembrane potential is – 90 millivolts and post-burn cell membrane potential is altered to – 60 millivolts. This increase in potential is due to increase in intracellular sodium and hence increase in intracellular water which causes swelling of cells. These changes are reversed by adequate resuscitation because of restoration of activity of sodium pump which removes sodium and water from the cells.

There is also immediate hemolysis of red blood cells which varies with severity of burns. The effect of heat on red blood cells depends upon the amount of heat energy that has gone into the cells. There is complete destruction of RBC at the site of full thickness burns and the RBC's trapped in the capillaries. Further there is hemolysis of RBC because of direct exposure to heat and few of the RBC get deformed due to the heat and their life span is shortened. The first two are the immediate causes of anemia and the second is responsible for late anemia of burns.

Because of loss of plasma into extravascular space, there is hemoconcentration which is presented as rise in hematocrit or PCV (packed cell volume). This increases the viscosity of the blood which slows down the blood flow especially in the capillaries. In small burns, the loss of plasma is compensated by the physiological response in the body but in case of larger burns more than 15 percent TBSA in adults, the large plasma leak invariably leads to shock. This hypovolemia may be so profound that it decreases the perfusion of various organs of the body. The classical signs and symptoms of shock are restlessness, pallor, cold skin, tachycardia and low blood pressure. With early treatment these changes of shock can be prevented.

The plasma leak continues till the effected capillaries either get thrombosed because of increased viscosity of blood or they regain their normal permeability which takes about 18 72 hours.

Because of loss of normal function of skin in the burned areas, there is loss of water due to evaporation from the burn wound surface and it persists till the skin wounds heal. The formula used to estimate this fluid loss is:

$$\text{Evaporative water loss (ml/hr)}$$
$$= (25 + \% \text{ burns}) \times \text{BSA m}^2$$

We have simplified this calculation further— there is 20 times increase in the evaporation of water from the burn surface, therefore in a temperate climate with a patient sustaining 100 percent burns, his loss will be $500 \times 20 = 10,000$ ml (500 ml is normal evaporative loss from the skin in a temperate climate). It means for a 50 percent burns the evaporative water loss will be 5000 ml and for 25 percent burns, it will be 2500 ml.

The mobilization of edema fluid gradually increases following resuscitation but is variable because the loss of lymphatics in full thickness burns, fibrin deposition in burn edema and high CVP retard the edema resorption.

Lymphatics

Under normal conditions lymph is returned to the circulation. About 50 percent of total circulating plasma proteins escapes into interstitium daily which are carried away by the lymph vessels, thus re-expanding the vascular space. Following thermal injury, in 1 to 3 hours post-injury there is a 5 to 10 fold increase in lymph flow from the injured skin which returns the extravascular fluid back to the circulation. But the interstitial edema fluid forms a gel after 12 hours because of the leaked out proteins and fibrin deposition. This obstructs the local lymphatics and inhibits edema clearance. Resolution of edema depends upon restoration of lymphatic patency which takes a number of days to weeks.

Cardiovascular System

Is directly affected by the thermal injury because of the hypovolemia. The cardiac output falls by 40 to 60 percent because of:

- Loss of plasma which causes hypovolemia which causes decreased venous return
- Decrease in cardiac contractility
- Involvement of oxygen free radicals.

The continuous evaporative losses of fluid lead to hypertonic dehydration. The oxygen consumption is increased for a long period along with these losses. The hemolysis and formation of microthrombi cause a decrease in hemoglobin mass and decrease in oxygen carrying capacity of blood leading to hypoxia of tissues.

Endocrinal Response

The pituitary – adrenocortical axis undergoes activation after burns. Glucocorticoids stimulate protein catabolism. Aldosterone causes sodium retention in tissues and release of potassium with its loss in urine. The production of insulin in pancreas beta cells and glucagon in alpha cells is affected in burns. Later on there is resistance to insulin. The diminished tolerance to glucose results in hypoglycemia and glycosuria. Major burns results in dramatic increase in circulating catecholamines, cortisol and growth hormone. These hormones along with interleukin 1, stimulate mobilization of stored protein supporting host defence and recovery. The acute phase is mediated by cytokine interleukin I which increases amino acid, iron and zinc uptake and also increases protein synthesis.

Renal Function

Burns like any severe trauma affects the kidney function in many ways. Initially because of shock there is stimulation of renin angiotensin axis which tries to increase renal perfusion by vasoconstriction while increase in cellular damage from burns increases the load on the kidneys. Because of increased cell damage, there is increased urea formation and this increases excretory load on the kidney. Therefore, even with normal renal perfusion there may be raised blood urea. However, if there is no renal parenchymal damage, there will be no increase in serum creatinine value.

Because of increased load on the kidney in the post-burn phase which is further increased by bacterial septicemia there may be renal cellular damage which may be a part of multiorgan failure. In case of electrical burns because of muscle damage, there may be renal tubular damage and similarly in some chemical burns, there may be renal parenchymal damage and in these cases both blood urea and creatinine values rise. Renal failure diagnosed by oliguria or anuria with progressively rising blood urea and creatinine values towards the end of the first week is usually a part of multiorgan failure in patients with extensive burns which is usually due to gram-negative septicemia. This can be treated by controlling sepsis by appropriate antibiotics. Another cause for renal failure in later stages is usually drug induced nephrotoxicity which can be corrected by dose alteration or withdrawal of the drug if possible.

Immune Response

Thermal injury is associated with severe immuno-suppression because it affects the host defense mechanism. There are three types of normal host defence mechanisms. The first defence mechanism disrupted is the skin which acts as a mechanical barrier between the external and internal environment.

The second defence mechanism affected is the nonspecific vascular, cellular and humoral response which leads to release of inflammatory mediators and phagocytic cells which cause vascular stasis, sludging and thrombosis. This causes additional ischemia to tissues already damaged by the heat.

The third defense mechanisms of immune system affected by thermal injury are the T- cells and B- cells which are responsible for cellular immunity. The suppressor cells are increased and cellular immunity decreased after burns.

The persistent catabolic state and protein loss including loss of immunoglobulin through the burn wounds and decreased production of Ig G and Ig M antibodies also lead to suppression of this immunity.

CHAPTER 3

First Aid in Burns

There is no specific first aid in burns. The only first aid for burns is:

1. To put out the fire
2. Prevent increase in intensity of heat damage by fire.

The first action that needs to be taken when a person is suffering burns is to **PUT OUT THE FIRE**. This can be done in the following manner:

- *Douse the flames*: By making the patient lie supine as flames of the fire have a tendency to go upwards and if the patient keeps standing the flames of the fire cause further damage to the upper parts of the body whereas in lying down position the flames will go up and away from the body, thus avoiding damage to the other parts of the body. The flames have to be smothered by rugs, blanket or water or simply make the patient roll on the ground. The basic aim is (a) to cut off the fuel to the fire, i.e the oxygen supply is cut off by using banket and (b) cool the area affected by water. He /she is to be prevented from running as motion increases the flames and in upright position the flame and smoke cause more damage to facial area and also increases the incidence of inhalation injury.
- Remove hot liquids and chemicals from the site.
- Disconnect electrical supply.
- Use of water:The role of water in first aid for burns is limited. The earlier concept of "Pour water on Burns" is no longer true for all burns. Water is to be used only for dousing the fire. In superficial and localized small burns which are very painful, water acts as a soothing agent as it temporarily numbs the exposed

nerve endings. Tap water is very useful for this purpose. Irrigation of wounds with water can be used for 5 - 10 min only and not longer. It should not delay the transfer of patient to the hospital. Also in extensive burns prolong irrigation with water can lead to hypothermia and is therefore not advisable. Use of ice water is not advocated for pain relief in burns >15 percent as hypothermia caused by this can lead to ventricular fibrillation. Water is not to be used for dousing fire from electric burns.

- In chemical burns copious irrigation with water will dilute the concentration of the chemical and minimize the depth of damage. It is important to use running water to wash off the chemical and not immerse the body part in water as that might be more harmful because the chemical will continue to act on the part immersed in water in a vessel and also because some chemicals react with water leading to other side effects. Time should not be wasted in searching for specific neutralizing agents. Irrigation should be done till litmus test turns negative (for acid burns –if blue does not change to red it is an indication to stop irrigation and *vice versa* is true for alkali burns). In few chemical burns, water is contraindicated, e.g. heavy metals like sodium, potassium and calcium which react violently with water.

- In case of electric burns first electric supply is to be disconnected and patient to be removed from the source with the help of some insulated nonconducting material like wood or plastic thus ensuring that the rescuer is not electrocuted in the process of saving someones life. Following this, immediately the patients circulation and ventilation should be checked and CPR (cardiopulmonary resuscitation) to be started if in doubt, till specific treatment can be given.

- Clothing contaminated by burning agents should be removed and part covered with a clean cloth to prevent contamination. Salves and toothpaste and home remedies should not be applied to the burned areas as they may be difficult to remove when cleaning the area.
- Next the patient is to be shifted to a doctor who can assess and advise further treatment after assessing which patient requires OPD treatment and which patient requires to be admitted (as discussed in Table 1.1 :Chapter 1).

OPD Management

Criteria for OPD management:
- Burns < 15 percent BSA in adults
- Burns < 10 percent in children
- Full thickness burns < 2 percent.

Guidelines for OPD Treatment

- After thoroughly cleaning the burned surface with saline and removing all the loose epithelium, the wound is to be dressed with an antimicrobial agent or application of a biological dressing material.
- Tetanus toxoid injection is given to all patients if they are previously immunized but have not received TT in the last 5 years. If prior immunization is not documented or wound is severely contaminated,

Human tetanus immunoglobulin (TIG) should also be given(dose of 250 IU).

- Pain killer is to be given to reduce pain in superficial burns.
- Antibiotics have usually got no role to play in small or minor burns because they are sterile and if dressed properly there are no chances of wound infection.
- Patient is to be then sent home with clear instructions about contacting the doctor again in case of emergency which would be indicated if there is:
  — Fever with chills
  — Swelling or inability to use toes or fingers in limb burns
  — Pain increases
  — Foul smelling discharge
  — Increasing redness of skin around the wound.

In small burns the dressing can be changed every 3-5 days.

In Patient Management

Criteria for Hospital Admission

- All adults >15 percent BSA burns
- In children >10 percent burns
- Full thickness burns >2 percent
- Patient with diabetes or any other systemic illness
- Burns of face, perineum
- Inhalational injury
- Electrical injury
- Intoxicated patient with burns.

In all patients with moderate to severe burns there are signs and symptoms of some degree of shock in the form of chills, rigors, cold skin, dry tongue with feeling of thirst, restlessness, tachycardia and tachypnea. With early treatment these changes of shock can be prevented.

For all major and most moderate burns, patient needs to be kept first in the ICU (Fig. 3.1) where there are proper monitoring facilities. The airway and ventilation is to be assessed first especially in face burns or smoke inhalation. Oxygen is to be started in all such cases. If there is respiratory distress and ABG is abnormal, patient should be intubated.

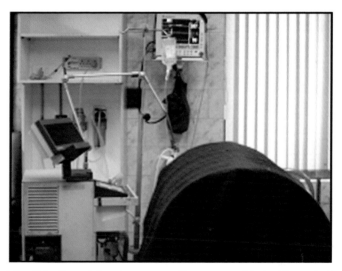

Fig. 3.1: Burn intensive care unit room provided with central noninvasive monitor, ventilator and wall mounted central suction and oxygen supply

IV fluids should be started immediately to restore circulation.

Wounds have to be dressed using some antimicrobial agent or biological dressings.

For pain management in major burns usually morphine or pethidine is given IV.

Tetanus immunization is to be given in the form of tetanus toxoid or TIG if indicated.

Use of antacids is also controversial. It was a standard teaching to give antacids prophylactically to avoid curling's ulcer (peptic ulcer). Usually Ranitidine 50 mg IV 8 hrly is given in adults or Pantaprazole 40 mg once a day. Though now it is believed that by giving antacids, the acid barrier is broken which allows translocation of bacteria across the gut.

Prophylactic antibiotics are not used in all admitted patients with major burns because the wounds are sterile at admission. Their use is to be restricted to only a few cases which will be discussed later.

Patient is to be kept in a warm environment where maintenance of room temperature and humidity is essential for treatment. All extensive burns are to be kept in a room with temperature $>26°C$ (26 - 32°C) and relative humidity 60 - 65 percent.

Definitive Assessment in a Burn Center

1. *Primary assessment*
   — Airway
   — Breathing
   — Circulation
   — Assess vitals

— Look for other life-threatening conditions (chest injury, cardiac complications, pneumothorax, etc)

2. *Secondary assessment*
   — Complete head to toe evaluation
   — Trauma other than burns(head injury or spinal injury in case of fall from height in electric burns)
   — Establish history of injury.

3. *Examine extremities for circumferential burns and pulses*

4. *Evaluate wounds – burn size and depth*

5. *Fluid resuscitation*

6. *Escharotomies if needed (Figs 3.2 to 3.10)*

7. *Evaluate airway and perform bronchoscopy if required*

8. *Laboratory tests.*

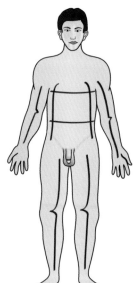

Fig. 3.2: Escharotomy incisions to chest, upper and lower limbs. Darts may be included to avoid linear scar contracture

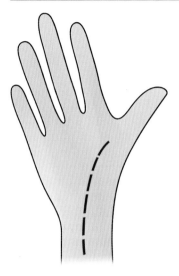

Fig. 3.3: Incision in palm to open carpal tunnel

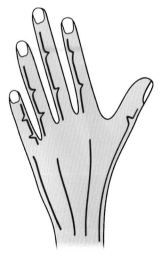

Fig. 3.4: Escharotomy incision on dorsum of hand

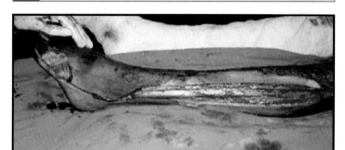

Fig. 3.5: Escharotomy incision converted to fasciotomy to release compartment pressure in lower leg

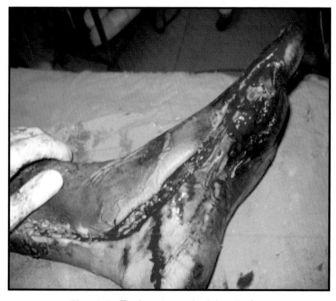

Fig. 3.6: Escharotomy incision in foot

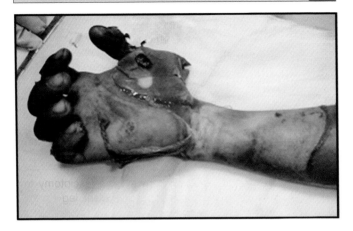

Fig. 3.7: Escharotomy incision in palm

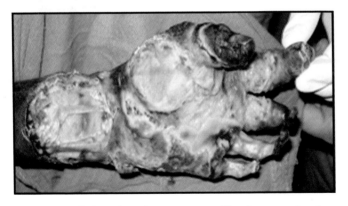

Fig. 3.8: Delayed escharotomy resulting in necrosis of digits and muscles

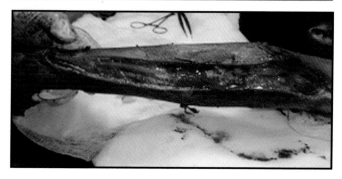

Fig. 3.9: Fasciotomy in forearm and arm medial side to release pressure completely

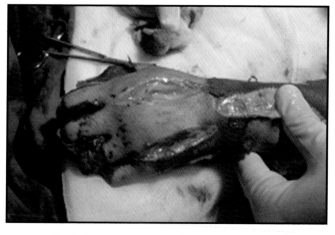

Fig. 3.10: Escharotomy incision on dorsum of hand showing the edematous tissues underneath

FLUID AND ELECTROLYTE REPLACEMENT

Loss of skin in burns results in increased water and heat loss. These losses are directly proportional to burn size. Large volume of fluid and electrolytes are lost from the burn surface and they need to be replaced during the first 12 to 24 hours to maintain circulatory volume and thus prevent acute renal failure. In burns <20 percent of BSA, fluids can be replaced orally but in > 20 percent burns in adults and > 10 percent in children, IV fluids are a must.

The ideal fluid for replacement is plasma because the fluid lost in the extravascular spaces in burns resembles plasma in its contents. But since plasma is not readily available, it is not the fluid of choice. Nevertheless patient requires colloid (like Dextran, Albumin, FFP, HPPF—Table 3.1) as replacement. The main advantage of using colloids are:

- Reduced volume of fluid required
- Maintains high urinary output and cardiac output
- Minimizes fluid loss into respiratory and gastrointestinal tract.

The disadvantage with colloids is that they are less effective due to leakage and increase the lung water in the second post-burn period.

Today's teaching is to give crystalloids because of their easy availability everywhere and economic feasibility.

Therefore in crystalloids (Table 3.2), the fluid of choice is *Ringer lactate* as it is a balanced electrolyte solution. The aim of fluid resuscitation is to have an alert, co-operative patient with a good urine output. There are several formulae used in different burns units all over the

Table 3.1: Colloid therapy		
Name	Formula	Timing
Harkins	100 ml plasma per 1% burn	In 24 hrs
Evans	1 ml plasma per 1% TBSA per kg wt. + 1 ml NS per 1% TBSA per kg wt.+ 2000 ml (daily requirement)	In 24 hrs
Brookes Army Hospital	0.5 ml plasma per kg wt/% TBSA +1.5ml RL per kg per% TBSA+2000 ml 5%dextrose	In 24 hrs
Slater	75 ml FFP /kg wt. +2 l RL	In 24 hrs
Muir and Barkley	Percent TBSA × wt./ 2 = ml of plasma in 4 hrs + 2400 ml dextrose	For two 4 hrly periods and then after these 12 hrs same volume in 6 hrs and 12 hrs.
Sorensen	120 ml/% TBSA Dextran 70	Half in first 8 hrs One fourth in next 16 hrs Rest one fourth in next 24 hrs

Table 3.2: Crystalloid therapy		
Name	Formula	Timing
Parkland Formula	4 ml /kg/% BSA RL	Half in first 8 hrs, half in next 16 hrs
Modified Brooke's Formula	1 ml /kg/% BSA of RL +2500 ml 5% D	Half in first 8 hrs and half in next 16 hrs
Hyperosmolar Solution Monafo's Formula	3.37 ml /kg/% BSA of hypertonic saline (This gives 0.7 mEq Na /kg/% BSA in 48 hrs)	In 48 hrs

world to calculate the fluid requirement. All patients need to be weighed prior to transfer to ward in order to calculate fluid requirement as all formulae are based on body weight and body surface area burned.

Hypertonic fluids –have the advantage of causing less edema and less risk of overloading as they decrease cardiac load and decrease the risk of respiratory complications. However, on the other hand they increase the risk of hypernatremia and hyperosmolality so they are not favored.

There is a very simple formula for calculating fluid requirement in burns (which is true for colloids), i.e. for every 10 percent of TBSA in adults, 1 to 1½ liters of fluid is required whereas in children, for every 15 percent TBSA, one plasma volume of fluid is required.

Though the most common formula used is Parkland formula or Modified Brook's formula. In subsequent 24 hours, evaporative losses from burned surface are replaced at 1 ml/kg/percent burn daily and in this colloids are given in a volume of 0.3 - 0.5 ml/kg/percent burn to correct plasma volume. The rate is adjusted hourly to get urine output of 0.5 ml/kg/hr. Potassium replacement is to be given only after 3 days post-burn because for the first 48 hrs the body compensates for the losses.

Fluid requirement in children is different from adults because there is a variability in BSA and weight in a growing child. Also, because of small glycogen stores, infants require glucose since they are prone to hypoglycemia in the initial resuscitation period. Therefore basal maintenance fluid in the form of 5 percent glucose containing solution is required. Also children are easily prone to hyponatremia which can cause cerebral edema and neuroconvulsive activity. Therefore daily maintenance fluid is given as a combination of 5 percent dextrose and saline in the form of N/3 or N/4 or N/5 DS. The most common formula used is Modified Brooke's formula, i.e 2 ml / kg / percent BSA + Daily requirement. Depending on weight and age, the daily requirement is calculated as follows:

- 100 ml / kg —— for first 10 kg
- 1000 ml + 50 ml / kg —— for 10- 20 kg
- 1500 ml + 25 ml / kg —— for > 20 kg

For type of fluid – in less than 2 months age – N/5 or N/6 DS:

- 2 months to 5 years age —— N/4 DS
- 5 to 12 years age —— N/4 or N/3 DS

All these formula only serve as a guide. More important is the response of the patient based on urine output. Additional fluids are needed in inhalational injury, electrical injury and delayed resuscitation cases.

Fluid requirement in patients with electrical burns is greater than in thermal burns because there is a danger of acute tubular necrosis and acute renal failure following precipitation of myoglobins from the dead tissue leading to myoglobinuria. This manifests as highly concentrated and pigmented urine. The aim in these patients is to maintain a higher urine output of 2 ml/kg/hr till the urine clears (water diuresis). Along with this, alkalization of urine by giving soda bi-carbonate and use of osmotic agents like mannitol is also helpful.

Monitoring

Urine Output

Though there are many new invasive and noninvasive methods available to monitor the resuscitation of a burn patient, the simplest and most practical method is to check the urine output on an hourly basis. An indwelling Foley's catheter should be placed to monitor urine output. A minimum urine output of 0.5 ml /kg /hr in adults and 1 ml /kg / hr in children should be maintained to ensure adequate resuscitation. This is an accurate method for monitoring burn resuscitation in majority of the cases. But it is not accurate for patients with endocrine problems or cardiovascular disorders. In those patients invasive methods will be more ideal.

Invasive Methods

These include:
- CVP monitoring
- Swanz Ganz catheterization
- Cardiac output measurement.

However, these invasive techniques are more useful in complicated and extensive burns.

The other vitals to be monitored are (Fig. 3.11)
- Peripheral pulses
- Blood pressure
- Respiratory rate
- Heart rate
- Temperature

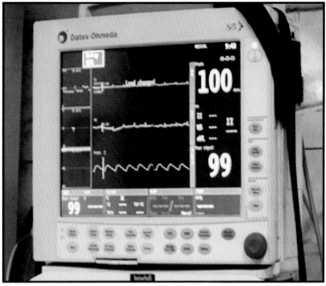

Fig. 3.11: Noninvasive monitor displaying all the vitals of the patient

Enteral Feeding

The earlier teaching was to keep the patient nil orally, as extensive burns were associated with severe splanchnic vasoconstriction in order to maintain systemic circulation. In this situation if the patient takes orally there is a likelihood of vomiting because of ileus. However, prolonged splanchnic vasoconstriction may cause ischemic necrosis of gut leading to perforation and bleeding. Therefore, nowadays it is recommended that enteral feeds with clear fluids is started on admission along with IV fluids and not to give more than one fourth of daily requirement in first 24 hours. With improvement in systemic circulation, oral feeds are gradually increased till full normal daily requirement is reached. IV fluids are then reduced at the same rate so as to just cover for the evaporative losses. After 24 hours, ideally majority of the fluid requirement should be provided by enteral route.

Laboratory Investigations

1. Laboratory investigations are an integral part of burn management. Initially following burn injury there are both hematological and biochemical changes. For proper fluid resuscitation, hematocrit is a very vital indicator of resuscitation as hemoconcentration indicates hypovolemia. In initial stages when the fluid therapy is just started, the hemoglobin and PCV are both raised but by 48 hours when the resuscitation is completed the levels come back to normal. So it should be estimated one hourly initially, followed by 4 hourly and then daily estimation till the level returns to normal.
2. A complete hemogram should be performed daily.
3. Since electrolyte changes are inevitable, sodium and potassium levels should be estimated once daily.
4. Kidney and liver function tests should be monitored daily for the first week followed by weekly tests till the patient recovers.
5. Other tests include:
   — Chest X-ray
   — ECG
   — Blood sugar(depending on patients age)—These should be done to have a baseline study.

6. All burn patients should have their throat and nasal swab taken daily for culture and wound swab for culture and sensitivity after 48 hours.

7. Role of routine blood culture in burns is controversial. It does not have much significance in case of gram-negative burn wound sepsis, because in these cases there is a release of toxins by the gram-negative organisms, present in the burn wound, into the blood stream. So that there will be no growth of these bacteria in the blood culture. But in cases where there is invasive sepsis in which the organisms invade the bloodstream from the wound or from the patient's own gut or respiratory tract, etc blood culture will be positive.

CHAPTER 4

Acute Burn Wound Management

The aim of local wound management is to (a)prevent wound from getting colonized with bacteria and then leading to systemic invasion and sepsis and (b)decrease evaporative losses. After cleaning thoroughly with saline, the loose necrotic epithelium is removed and wound is to be dressed.

Management of blister (Figs 4.1A and B): It is a very controversial topic.It is believed that the blister fluid contains plenty of prostaglandin E which prevents pain. So some people believe that if burns are not extensive and blisters are small (<5 cm) and multiple, they can be left as such. Also because the devitalized epithelium of the blisters acts as a protective cover over the underlying viable epithelium. Bullae on palm of hand are firm and can be left as such to serve as a temporary dressing. But in case of extensive burns with big (>5 cm) and thin blisters or blisters which are broken need to be dealt with because the chances of their bursting accidentally and fluid getting contaminated and later infected increases the chances of invasive wound sepsis. So we believe that in these cases it is better to incise the blister, drain out all the fluid and remove the dead epithelium of the roof so that there can be no recollection of fluid. Some believe that the dead epithelial layer acts as a temporary dressing to the underlying wound but it is seen that if this layer is left over the healthy epithelium, it never adheres to it and the surface is always wet which increases the chances of infection. So it is considered better to deroof all the blisters completely and the area is then dressed with some topical antimicrobial agent.

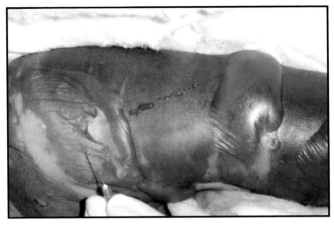

Fig. 4.1A: Superficial dermal burns with blisters. Blister is incised with needle the fluid is evacuated and roof epithelium of the blister removed

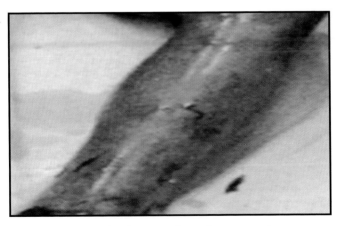

Fig. 4.1B: Same patient after removal of blisters and loose skin

Wound dressing:

Any dressing used for burns should fulfill the following criteria:

- It should be nonadherent
- It should prevent growth of bacteria
- It should prevent evaporative losses from the burn wound
- It should promote epithelialization of the wound.

The risk of wound contamination can be decreased by using:

a. Topical antimicrobial agents
b. Biological or synthetic skin substitutes.

After cleaning the surface of the burn wound, paraffin gauze is applied over it,over which an antimicrobial cream is applied, followed by gauze and then gamgee. A gentle compressive bandage is then tied over this (Fig. 4.3). Small wound dressing can be changed in 3-5 days.In extensive burns dressing may need to be changed more frequently depending on the soakage and smell.In some centers it is preferred to treat burn wounds by exposure method. In these cases an antimicrobial cream is applied over the wounds and they are left open (Figs 4.2A and B).This, however, increases evaporative losses and chances of cross infection. Face is usually left exposed because infection is very rare in this vascular area and the healing is also quick. Hand burns are dressed and their position fixed in a functional position so as to prevent contractures. Or after application of antibacterial cream, the hands are covered with a plastic bag to allow active physiotherapy.

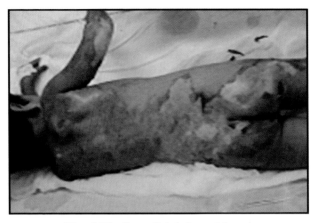

Fig. 4.2A: Superficial dermal burns
on back due to scalds in a child

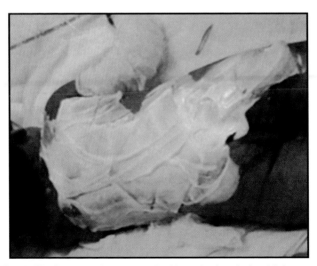

Fig. 4.2B: Same patient treated with topical antimicrobial cream
(1% Silver sulphadiazine)—applied as a thick layer –1cm thick
layer—Exposed method of treating burn wound

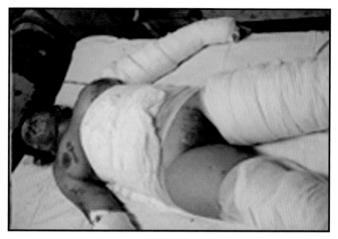

Fig. 4.3: Closed method of treating burn wound

TOPICAL ANTIMICROBIAL AGENTS

Normally speaking, all fresh burn wounds are sterile because the heat kills all the surface pathogens. The antimicrobial agents are used for inhibiting bacterial colonization of the burn wounds, thus preventing conversion of superficial burns to deep burns. Thus applied in the initial dressing, they play a prophylactic role.

Criteria for Ideal Antimicrobial Agent

- It should be effective against broad group of organisms.
- Easy and painless to apply.
- Capable of good penetration of wound without itself getting absorbed systemically thus avoiding any systemic toxicity.

- If at all absorbed, it should be metabolized and excreted in a short time.
- Organisms should not develop resistance to the agent.

There are various agents used for this purpose. The commonly used ones are:

1% SILVER SULFADIAZINE

It is the most commonly used agent for burn dressing and also the most effective in terms of antibacterial control, patient comfort and compliance and is used for closed dressings. Is to be applied as a thick layer.

Advantages

It is highly effective against gram-negative bacteria especially pseudomonas because it delays colonization. It is also effective against gram-positive organism and *Candida albicans* and herpes virus.

It can be applied easily and action lasts for 24 hours. There is minimal pain during its application and is non-staining.

Tissue penetration is moderate.

Can be used for both open and closed dressings.

Disadvantages

Causes transient leukopenia which resolves on its own so there is no need to stop its application.

If dressing is removed after 2 or 3 days, formation of a thin pseudoeschar is seen over the wound which can be removed by gentle debridement.

SILVER NITRATE SOLUTION

Is used as a 0.5 percent solution. It is bacteriostatic and has to be applied every 2 hours to keep the dressing wet so as to keep the concentration of the solution < 2 percent (which is caustic and cytotoxic). Since it is prepared in distilled water, its 0.5 percent solution is hypotonic.

Advantages

It is effective against a wide bacterial spectrum as well as fungal organism.
It is bacteriostatic.
It is minimally absorbed from burn wound so no signs of toxicity are seen.
Its application is painless.

Disadvantages

It has limited tissue penetration.
Its application causes black staining of skin and clothes. Because of the hypotonicity of the solution, it can cause substantial leaching of sodium, potassium and other plasma solutes from the burn wound, leading to hypochloremia and hyponatremia especially in infants and children. Therefore serum electrolytes have to be monitored.
The nitrate component can be reduced to nitrite by some gram-positive and gram-negative organisms which when absorbed can cause methemoglobinemia.

MAFENIDE ACETATE OR SULFAMYLON

It is used in 10 percent concentration and as a thick layer over the wound. Has to be applied twice daily, i.e. every 12 hours.

Advantages

It has potent antibacterial action.
Very good penetration of burn eschar and also efficient penetration of cartilage. Therefore it is best used for burned ears and nose. Because of its excellent penetration, it is more useful for established burn wound infection and not for routine use.

Disadvantages

Application is very painful due to its high osmolarity.
May produce metabolic acidosis because it has carbonic anhydrase inhibiting property, leading to alkaline diuresis.
It can lead to acid base abnormality if used in > 20 percent burns.

Framycetin (Soframycin)

Is very useful for small areas.

Disadvantages

If used liberally in extensive burns, its absorption can lead to renal toxicity.

Gentamicin

Since this is used systemically, its use as a topical agent will increase the chances of hypersensitivity reactions.

Disadvantages

Its systemic absorption can lead to nephrotoxicity and ototoxicity

Chlorhexidine and Povidone Iodine

Though they have a broad spectrum of action, they have only limited use because of their use in small burns only. If used in larger areas they get absorbed and lead to hepatic and renal toxicity. Chlorhexidine is painful to apply also.

Furacin (Nitrofurazone)

Has bactericidal action against both gram-negative and gram-positive organisms.

Advantages

It penetrates rapidly through eschar.
There is low resistance to this agent.
Use is restricted for MRSA infection of burn wound.

Disadvantages

It is not effective against pseudomonas.
Causes discomfort on application.
Can cause renal failure on systemic absorption if used in large amounts.

BIOLOGICAL DRESSINGS

Biological dressings can be natural or synthetic.
   Amniotic membrane is a very useful natural dressing material except for the following disadvantages:
• Predelivery HIV and HBsAg is to be done
• To be procured from the obstetrics department
• Storage problem
• Prefer cesarean-section amniotic membrane.

Xenograft: is graft obtained from animal skin. Usually porcine skin is a favourite amongst burn surgeons in the developed countries because of its availability even though it is expensive. In our country it is not used because of its nonavailabiltiy.

Collagen Dressings

There are various other collagen based dressings available for temporary wound closure. Collagen is the basic constituent of connective tissue in the skin and is mainly type I. Collagen is extracted from bovine source or sheep intestine. These can be either wet or dry variety. There are many commercial preparations for each of these. Wet collagen (available as Kollagen) has a higher reaction rate because of the preservative especially in children in the form of febrile reaction. Dry collagen (Skin temp —Fig. 4.4, Healicoll) has a very low antigenicity because it is gamma irradiated.

Advantages

* They seal the wound thus avoiding contamination and infection.
* Decrease the evaporative losses.
* Non-adherent and conforms well to the surface.
* Painless application and removal.
* Decreases pain and discharge both.
* These are very useful in superficial partial thickness and deep partial thickness burns as they promote healing because of the above factors.

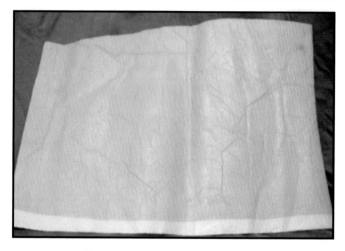

Fig. 4.4: Dry collagen (skin temp)

Application of Collagen Sheets (Figs 4.5A to 4.7C)

After cleaning the wound with saline, collagen sheet is applied directly to the wound. Wet collagen has to be thoroughly washed with saline as well. This may be covered with 1 percent SSD and then a secondary dressing. Collagen dressings need not be changed very frequently. Usually there is little soakage only so the dressing need not be changed before 4-5 days. Both the frequency and number of dressing decrease with their use. During change of dressing only the outer non absorbable sheet is peeled off as the collagen is generally absorbed. The

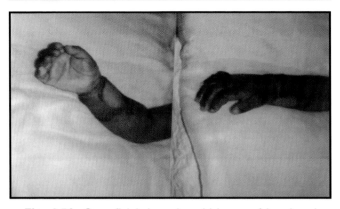

Fig. 4.5A: Superficial dermal scald burns of hand and forearm of a child

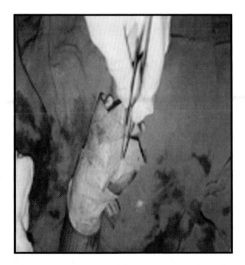

Fig. 4.5B: Dry collagen (skin temp) dressing applied to same patient as a first dressing —child was very comfortable with no pain or discharge

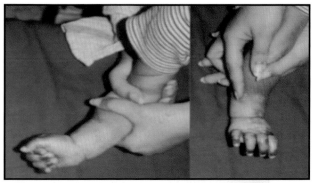

Fig. 4.5C: Completely healed wounds after 8 days—required only two dressing changes

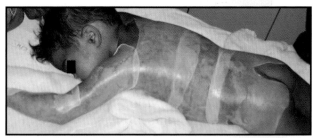

Fig. 4.6A: Superficial and deep dermal burns on back, buttocks and arm of a child with wet collagen dressing

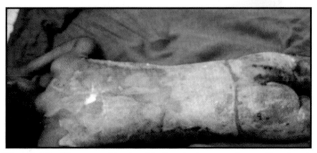

Fig. 4.6B: Same patient with healed wounds on the back and only small raw areas over buttocks

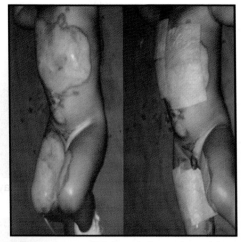

Fig. 4.7A: Mixed superficial and deep dermal burns being dressed with dry collagen

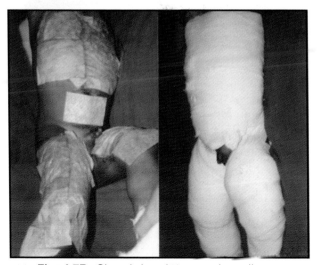

Fig. 4.7B: Closed dressing over dry collagen

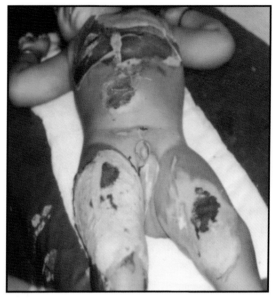

Fig. 4.7C: Same patient after 15 days showing collagen adherent to areas of superficial dermal burns and absorbed in areas of deep dermal burns

area is cleaned and another sheet reapplied. This technique is painless unlike the usual dressing.

CHAPTER 5

Late Burn Wound Management

There are various modes of handling burn wounds:

1. Conservative treatment
   - Dressings with topical antimicrobial agents
   - Dressings followed by secondary grafting of granulating wounds.

   This treatment is mainly indicated for superficial and superficial dermal burns.It may also be indicated for deep dermal and full thickness burns where immediate excision and grafting is not possible.

2. Early excision and grafting ⎫ Indicated for deep
3. Late excision and grafting   ⎬ dermal and full
4. Progressive debridement   ⎭ thickness burns

All these techniques can be used in different patients or different areas of the same patient. The main aim of treatment is to cover the burn wound as soon as possible by the most suitable method available depending on the specific wounds. A number of skin substitutes have been used but no substitute works better than skin itself for wounds which will not heal on their own. Biological dressings are useful in gaining time till the wounds can be grafted in case of extensive wounds all of which cannot be grafted in a single stage.

SURGICAL MANAGEMENT OF BURN WOUNDS

Amongst the recent advances in burn management is the surgical treatment of the burn wounds (Fig. 5.1). The conservative management of burn wounds by dressings followed by secondary grafting has been taken over by early surgical management of the burn wounds, especially in case of deep dermal and full thickness burns. Though this is an aggressive approach it has several advantages over the conservative management techniques.

Advantages

1. Fastens the healing process thus decreasing morbidity and pain.
2. Decreases the hospital stay.
3. Problems of infection and nutrition seen in chronic burn wounds are circumvented.
4. Contractures if formed are less severe.

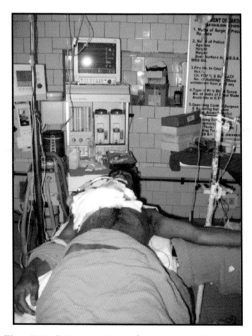

Fig. 5.1: Fully equipped burns operating room

5. Cosmetic appearance of grafted skin is better than wounds healing by hypertrophic scarring or contractures.
6. Mortality and morbidity in cases of early excision appears to be less than those who are managed conservatively.

Types of Burn Wound Excision

The burn wound excision may be broadly classified into:

1. *Primary excision*: It is done within 3 - 7 days following burns. It is actually a delayed primary excision because it is done after the third day of burns for extensive burns. This is further subclassified into Tangential, Sequential and Fascial excision, depending upon the technique used.

2. *Delayed primary excision*: It is done after 2 - 3 weeks of conservative management of burn wound by dressings with topical antimicrobial agents. This is in those cases of deep dermal burns in whom primary excision is not done and it is found that the dead layer of upper dermis is still adherent to the underlying live reticular dermis.

3. *Secondary excision*: This is basically a procedure for preparing the wound bed for grafting by removing the eschar. It is synonymous with surgical toilet or debridement.

Types of Primary Excision

1. *Tangential excision*: It is used typically for deep dermal burns. In this technique, the wound is excised with

Humby's knife till healthy viable dermis over which skin graft is applied.

2. *Sequential excision*: It is also used for deep burns in which Humby's knife is used to sequentially excise all necrotic tissue until viable tissue is encountered which can be either viable deep dermis or viable fat or fascia. This area is also immediately grafted. This technique is most effective for mixed deep dermal and partial thickness burns in which sequential excision will help in saving the viable dermis or fat which would otherwise be sacrificed if the entire burned area were to be removed with a surgical blade.

3. *Suprafascial full thickness excision*: It is indicated for full thickness burn wounds.In this the full thickness of burned skin with subcutaneous tissue is excised with a surgical knife till the deep fascia.This can be immediately grafted because fascia is a healthy bed for graft uptake.

4. *Subfascial excision*: It involves excising till below the deep fascia, thus reaching the muscles. Though in these cases the chances of graft take is poorer compared to suprafascial excision.

5. *Escharectomy and delayed skin grafting*: This was practiced earlier for partial and full thickness burns in which the apparently nonviable eschar is excised with a skin grafting knife till minimal bleeding bed is encountered. This is then covered with a biological dressing and reassessed after 48 - 72 hours to see for remaining dead tissue, which is again excised and dressed till healthy granulation tissue appears. This is then secondarily grafted. This procedure is between

primary excision and secondary grafting following conservative management of burn wounds as it takes 7 - 10 days for the granulation tissue to appear following excision of dead tissue. This is, however, not practiced anymore. It is suitable for cases in which primary excision cannot be done due to medical reasons or associated injuries.

ANATOMICAL AND PHYSIOLOGICAL BASIS FOR EXCISION

The principal and type of excision can be explained by the anatomy of skin and depth of burn. For excision purpose the depth of burns is broadly classified into superficial and deep burns. Superficial burns involve the epidermis and upper half of dermis and these heal without intervention in 10 days. Deep burns are those which involve the entire epidermis and dermis and these do not heal on their own and require surgical intervention. In between these two are deep dermal burns which involve the epidermis and two thirds of dermis and these heal in a long time with severe hypertrophic scarring and contracture formation. So in these cases if tangential excision is done it would not only improve morbidity but even mortality is reduced dramatically. The deep dermis may be anatomically dead but physiologically viable, therefore it needs to be covered with split skin graft following excision.

Guidelines for Primary Excision

- *Extent of excision*: Burn excision should not be taken lightly as the surgical procedure causes further stress on the body which is already highly stressed out by the burn injury. Normally at any given time surgical excision of > 15 percent TBSA requires high degree of medical and surgical care. Where these facilities are not available,one must avoid excision in extensive burns. Some areas which can safely be excised under tourniquet like upper and lower limbs, can be taken up for surgery.

- Age is no criteria as such for excision except that it is not usually done for infants and toddlers because of technical difficulty during excision caused by the abundant adipose tissue and thin skin. Very old patients (> 60 years) are not preferred because of associated medical problems.

- *Type of burn*: Usually hot water scalds and flash burns are not excised because they heal on their own. Electrical burn, alkali burns and hot molten metal burns are taken up for primary excision.

- Area of body involved affects the decision for surgery because usually the flat surfaces of evenly contoured areas are taken up for tangential excision like extremities, chest, abdomen, scalp. Face and perineum are difficult areas for tangential excision.

- Contraindications for excision - associated inhalational injury:
  - Any systemic disorders including dysfunction, renal, hepatic or cardiac dysfunction
  - Impaired coagulation profile.

- *Timing for primary excision*: Usually done between 3rd and 5th day following burns. Rationale for not doing it before 3rd day is to give adequate time for resuscitation especially in extensive burns and to avoid unnecessary excision of deeper tissues which may otherwise revascularize after resuscitation is completed. Excision is not done after 5 days because by then there is significant bacterial colonization of wound which will inhibit graft uptake. Beyond 7 days there is softening of the surface of wound which makes excision technically difficult.

- Extent of excision is usually limited to 15 percent TBSA in one sitting. In case of extremities where tourniquet is used, this can be increased to 30 percent TBSA also.
- *Area of excision*: Usually the trunk is preferred for first sitting of excision because it is easy to excise in this area. In females, lower limb are excised first.
- Preoperative investigation:
  - Hemoglobin and PCV — to assess for adequate resuscitation
  - Serum electrolytes — to ensure that sodium and potassium values are within normal range
  - Kidney function test
  - Total serum protein
  - Platelet count
  - TLC, DLC
  - Culture of wound is very important as the only contraindication for any excision is the growth of beta hemolytic streptococcus.
- Preoperative prophylactic antibiotics are to be started covering streptococcus and staphylococcus.
- Adequate blood to be arranged for surgery. Generally one unit blood is required for every 5 percent TBSA excised.
- Preoperative mapping of areas to be excised is done delineating clearly the areas of deep dermal burns from

the areas of superficial dermal burns by capillary refilling and sensation. Partial thickness burns which blanch on pressure with prompt refilling and are sensitive to pinprick will heal in 3 weeks and therefore should not be excised. Areas which are insensate and show no capillary refilling with no signs of involvement of deeper structures are the ideal areas for tangential excision.

Technique of tangential excision (Figs 5.2A to 5.3C): First the areas of deep dermal burns are marked or mapped as per the clinical assessment. For tangential excision with Watson's modification of Humby's knife, the knife is set to take thick split skin graft. Saline is used to keep the area wet and help in easy movement of knife. Slices of burned tissue are excised till viable tissue with brisk bleeding is encountered. Viable dermis appears shiny white in color with multiple bleeding points. To avoid sudden large volume of blood loss, one smaller area is excised and perfect hemostasis is achieved before starting excision over another area. Topical adrenaline solution for 5-10 minutes and then use of slow water jet over excised area to localize bleeding points for bipolar cauterization are commonly used to achieve hemostasis. Exposed viable dermis and other tissue are covered immediately by adrenaline solution soaked sponges to avoid its desiccation.

Smaller areas of burn surrounded by unburnt skin are difficult to excise by large size knife. Hence, smaller knives like silver knife is used. For harvesting graft from uneven areas like chest wall and scalp, it is advisable to inject saline in subcutaneous tissue.

To reduce blood loss during excision from the burned areas over extremities, tourniquet is inflated 100 mm Hg

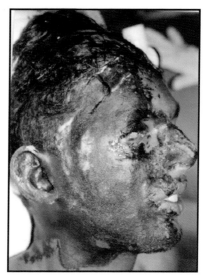

Fig. 5.2A: Deep dermal acid burns of face

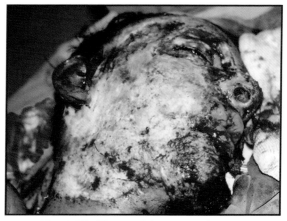

Fig. 5.2B: Tangential excision for face
showing viable bleeding dermis

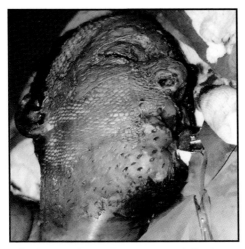

Fig. 5.2C: Skin grafting of same area following excision

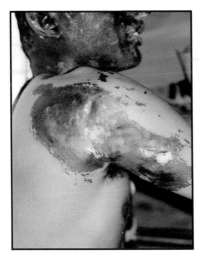

Fig. 5.2D: Deep dermal acid burns over shoulder

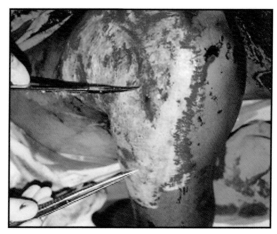

Fig. 5.2E: Tangential excision of same areas showing excision done till viable reticular dermis which is shiny white with multiple bleeding points

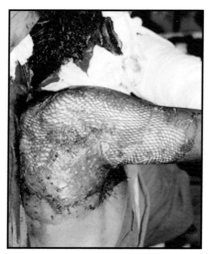

Fig. 5.2F: Split skin graft applied to the excised areas

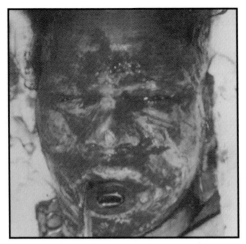

Fig. 5.3A: Tangential excision of face

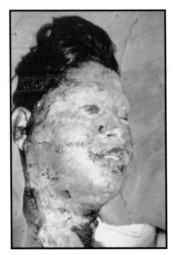

Fig. 5.3B: Nonmeshed graft applied to the areas as per aesthetic units

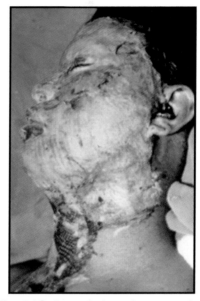

Fig. 5.3C: Lateral view of same patient

above systolic pressure. After excision is complete topical epinephrine solution may be used for 10 minutes before release of the tourniquet. After release of the tourniquet, the limb is again wrapped in epinephrine solution soaked gauze for another 5 minutes.

For assessment of viability of the tissue after excision under tourniquet and epinephrine solution, appearance of the left tissue is observed: The dermis must be pearly white, with no hemorrhagic staining; minor vessels on the wound surface must be patent; the fat must be pale yellow, firm, and moist (dry, or golden brown fat is unhealthy); and the excised wound rapidly becomes hyperemic, even under tourniquet control. In particular, shortly after what appears to be adequate excision, the white dermis and pale yellow fat appear to develop hemorrhagic staining. Although this usually represents re-perfusion, it can easily be confused with the staining that characterizes thermally injured tissue. Thus, there may be a tendency to unnecessarily re-excise the area. Hence, the level of excision is most easily determined with the initial passes of the debriding blade, and should not be altered thereafter unless there is convincing evidence of inadequate excision (e.g. tissue fails to re-perfuse, remains dry, or contains thrombosed vessels on the wound surface).

Advantages: As compared to excision en-block, tangential excision produces less contour problems and better cosmetic result. This technique results in better texture of grafted skin and greater sensitivity.

Complications: The most important complication is bleeding from the excised wounds specially in areas where tourniquet cannot be applied. Next is failure of graft take, which may be due to inadequate excision, infection, hematoma, lack of proper immobilization.

Postoperative Management

In immediate postoperative period hemoglobin, PCV, serum electrolyte level is done to assess blood loss and appropriate action is taken as per report. Hourly vital signs and urine output is measured and intravenous fluid is administered as per requirement. Antibiotics, as per culture and sensitivity report, analgesic and supportive treatment is instituted. Depending on GI function, oral feeding is started after 6 hours or later.

Depending on wound condition, dressing is usually done on 5th day and then depending on the graft take. As one usually expects a 100 percent graft uptake, two or three dressings may be required after first dressing till the area is totally dry. Donor area heals in 10-14 days. Physiotherapy is started after 7 days. Any splint if required is delivered at the time of discharge or during follow-up visits.

DELAYED BURN WOUND GRAFTING

Guidelines for Grafting

- The primary requirement for grafting of wound bed is a clean wound devoid of necrotic tissue with healthy granulation tissue or vascularized bed for nourishment of overlying graft.
- If granulation tissue is infected and dirty it should be treated first by local dressings and systematic antibiotics if quantitative count is $> 10^5$ org/ gm of tissue (Figs 5.4A to C).
- If bed shows hypergranulating tissue, prior dressings with hypertonic saline is useful.
- Immobilization of part in order to avoid shearing of graft with wound bed is required.
- The priority areas for skin coverage should be mapped out so as to cover them first in order to give good aesthetic as well as good functional result. These areas include face, neck, hands, elbows, axilla and knee joints. If the face and neck is covered early, contractures in neck and lip area are prevented thus avoiding intubation problems in surgeries later on.
- If major joint areas are covered the patient can be mobilized early with minimal functional restrictions.
- Grafts applied to aesthetic units should not be meshed.

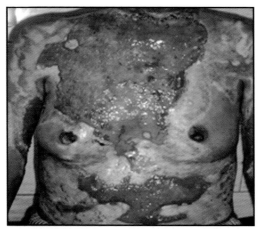

Fig. 5.4A: Unhealthy pale hypergranulating post-burn raw areas from deep burns, not fit for grafting. These areas require blood transfusion to build up the hemoglobin and frequent dressings with hypertonic saline to improve the areas

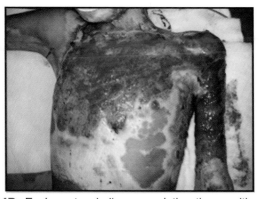

Fig. 5.4B: Exuberant red slimy granulation tissue with scanty discharge, though giving a false impression of healthy granulation because of its red look, is indicative of staphylococcal infection. Requires topical anti-staphylococcal treatment as well as systemic antibiotics effective against staphylococcus to prepare the wound

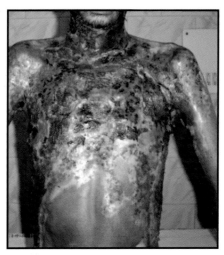

Fig. 5.4C: Successful split skin grafting of the same area as in Figure 5.4B after proper preparation of the wounds

- Post-burn raw areas essentially require thin grafts because:
  a. Take of thin grafts is better.
  b. Donor areas heal early with minimal scarring.
  c. In extensive burns with limited normal skin, these limited donor areas can be reused again and again for procuring grafts.
  d. Donor site morbidity is reduced.

Classification of Grafts According to Donor

1. *Autograft:* is the patient's own skin which is best used to cover the wounds. The best donor site is the patients thighs or upper arm. But in case of extensive burns

these areas can be reused to obtain grafts again after 2 weeks because usually thin grafts are taken. In case the area is extensive, scalp is a good donor site because it can be reused many times as a donor area.

2. *Homograft:* It is obtained from any other human being except the patient himself. Usually the patients own relatives are chosen as donors. The best being siblings and next the parents. However, fresh cadaveric skin can also be used if prior permission has been taken. In such donors, HIV and HBsAg is tested prior to donation as the contraindications for homograft use is hepatitis, AIDS and disseminated fungal infections. Usually fresh skin is used but skin stored for less than 2 weeks can also be used. Older skin can be used in early phases of wound debridement and preparation for auto grafting. A good 'Take' of homograft is a good test for wound readiness to accept auto graft (Figs 5.5A to D).

3. *Heterograft/ Xenograft:* It is graft obtained from another species. Usually porcine skin is used. Though used very rarely because it is very expensive.

4. *Isograft:* It is graft harvested from an identical twin. There is no rejection of this graft.

The turning point in burn patient management is the time when all his wounds are covered with skin - whether it is homograft or autograft or heterograft.

TYPES OF GRAFT

1. *Pinch graft:* It is a small piece of skin about 5 mm in diameter which is harvested by elevating the skin with a sharp needle and cutting a pyramid shaped

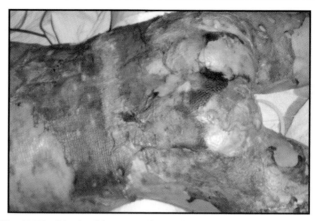

Fig. 5.5A: Meshed homograft applied to extensive post-burn raw areas in a child as a temporary cover. Shows good take of graft

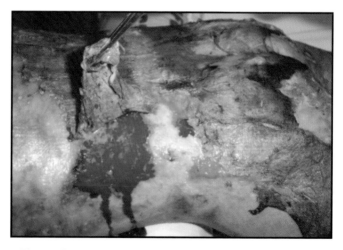

Fig. 5.5B: Homograft being removed after 5 -7days and underlying bed healthy and fit for grafting

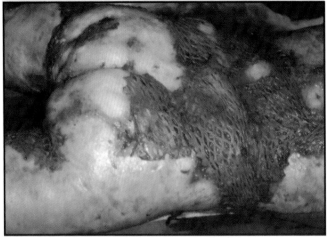

Fig. 5.5C: Same wounds autografted

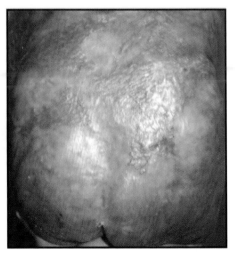

Fig. 5.5D: Completely healed areas
2 weeks after autografting

piece of epidermis and dermis. Is not practiced anymore for burn wounds because it gives a poor cover.

2. *Stamp grafts:* are square or rectangle shaped pieces of split thickness grafts which are placed on the wound with gaps in between the stamps which get covered by proliferation of epithelial cells from the margins of the grafts. Their use in burn wound coverage is very rare now with the use of Humby's knife and dermatome.

3. *Sheet grafts:* are the most widely used for covering burn wound because of use of Humby's knife and dermatome. Grafts obtained by this method can be
   a. Thin – 0.006 to 0.008 inch
   b. Intermediate – 0.008 to 0.014 inch
   c. Thick – 0.014 to 0.021 inch

4. *Meek grafts:* are being used lately. It is a kind of stamp grafting though in this procedure sheets of grafts are first procured which are then applied on a sheet with dermis up and then passed through a machine which divides the graft into small pieces or stamps. This sheet is then stretched so that the pieces of graft get separated by 2-3 mm and then applied as such on the raw areas. This method is preferred in extensive burns where the donor areas are very limited.

Advantage of Grafting

1. Negative nitrogen balance is minimized
2. Evaporative losses are decreased
3. Patient shifts from catabolic state to anabolic state
4. Patient becomes pain free

5. General condition improves dramatically
6. Dramatic decrease in bacterial count in granulation tissue under skin grafts after 24 hours.

TECHNIQUE FOR SPLIT SKIN GRAFTING

In the operation theater, under anesthesia, the skin is harvested with either a hand held Humby's knife (Fig. 5.6) or a electric or pneumatic dermatome from the lower limb, trunk and upper limb circumferentially. Usually for a burn wound a thin to medium thickness skin graft (0.015 inch thick) is most easy to manipulate and apply to the wounds (Fig. 5.7A). If thick graft is harvested, the skin tends to shrink, edges roll up and it does not lie flat on recipient area. Also the donor area takes a longer time to heal and cannot be used for reharvesting a graft. At the same time these donor area scars tend to hypertrophy later on. Give 2 - 3 weeks time between recropping of a certain donor site when thin graft is taken initially. If skin graft is taken from uneven surfaces like chest or abdomen, the area can be infiltrated with saline to produce a smooth surface for harvesting graft with Humby's knife.

Broad and long sheets are preferred as they are easy to apply. These grafts are usually meshed either by hand (Fig. 5.7B) or a mesher (Figs 5.8 and 5.9). Meshing is done in the ratio of 1½ : 1 or 3 :1 depending on how much expansion is required which depends upon the requirement of graft. In face, meshing is not preferred. Advantage of meshing is not only to expand the graft but also allow drainage of blood and secretions and thus avoiding hematoma formation under the graft. The grafts are placed on the raw area without any sutures. The slits in the meshed graft should be placed parallel to the normal skin lines of the area to be grafted because this ensures minimal contraction and thus best cosmetic results.

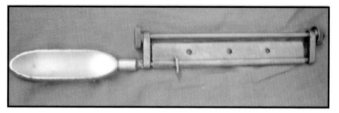

Fig. 5.6: Humby's skin grafting handle

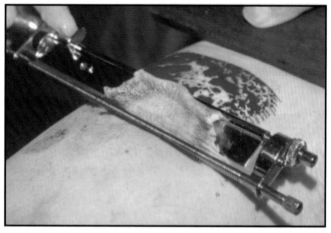

Fig. 5.7A: Split skin graft being harvested
by Humby's knife

Blood loss is an important factor during harvesting skin graft in a burn patient. The average blood loss in taking a split skin graft is 23 ml/100 cm^2 of donor area. So accordingly blood should be arranged.

In the past any split skin graft used to be routinely covered with some occlusive dressing but over the years it has been seen that occlusive dressings are not necessary for

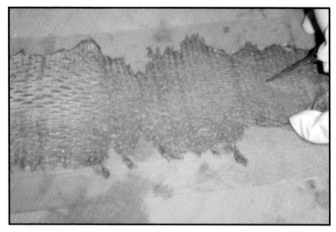

Fig. 5.7B: Hand meshing of split skin graft

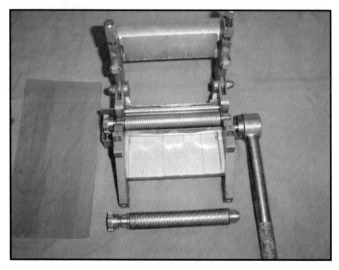

Fig. 5.8: Zimmer skin graft mesher. Skin graft can be expanded by 1.1, 1.5:1, 2:1, 3:1, 4:1 and 6:1 by using different blades

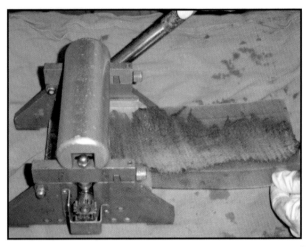

Fig. 5.9: Mesher in use. The skin graft is placed on a carrier which is passed through the mesher with extreme care so that the graft does not get rolled and entangled onto the blades

successful take of the graft. Infact that may even hinder the take because of friction between the dressing and graft bed especially in areas which cannot be immobilized for long like abdomen, chest, neckgroin, etc, because continuous movement of abdomen and chest with respiration produces shearing between the graft which is immobilized by dressing and the recipient area which is moving (Figs 5.10A and B).

In circumferential wounds of the limb, either a firm occlusive dressing is done or grafts are left exposed in case skeletal traction is used to elevate and immobilize the limb. If dressings are used as in case of extremities they have to be bulky enough to give sufficient compression as well as immobilization of extremity. A joint above and below the area grafted has to be immobilized to avoid movements completely so that there is no shearing of the graft.

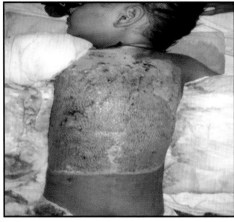

Fig. 5.10A: Six hours post-graft picture of meshed grafts placed on post-burn raw areas by exposed method, so that there is no friction between the graft and underlying wound because of movement of chest with respiration. Graft adherent to the surface as plasmatic imbibition has started

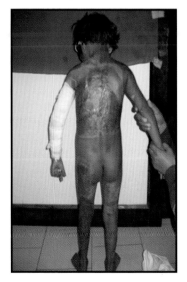

Fig. 5.10B: Completely healed grafted areas of same patient

Change of Dressing

Since all burn wounds are contaminated, it is advisable to change the first dressing after 48 - 72 hours postgraft because if delayed beyond this, purulent discharge may inhibit graft uptake. Second dressing change can be done at 4-5 days and then subsequently depending on 'take' of graft. Donor area dressing is to be opened only after 3 weeks, though if thin grafts have been harvested the donor areas heal in 2-3 weeks (Figs 5.14A to D).

HISTOLOGY OF SPLIT THICKNESS SKIN GRAFT UPTAKE (FIGS 5.11 TO 5.13)

Six hours post-graft: Graft nourishment starts by plasmatic imbibition and proliferation of host endothelium starts.

Twelve hours post-graft: Proliferated host endothelium starts penetrating the fibrin interface between graft and host.

Twenty-four hours post-graft: Neovascularization of graft by growth of host vessels begins.

Forty-eight hours post-graft: Vascular communication between graft and host is well established giving the graft a pink hue.

Three days post-graft: The epidermis of graft becomes thick and swollen with mitotic activity. Capillaries extend from the bed into the graft. Elastic fibres are normal in the graft and collagen is also normal in the bed.

One week post-graft: Epidermis is hyperplastic. Hair follicles disappear after heavy leukocytic infiltration. Elastic fibers get fragmented in the graft and in the bed also collagen fibers get dissolved.

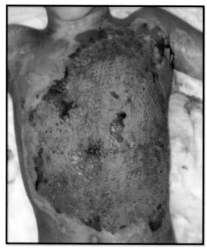

Fig. 5.11: Forty-eight hours after application of graft showing a pinkish hue which indicates neovascularization of graft has taken place

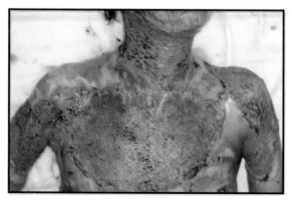

Fig. 5.12: Five days post-graft picture for extensive raw areas of chest, neck and upper arms showing 100 percent graft take

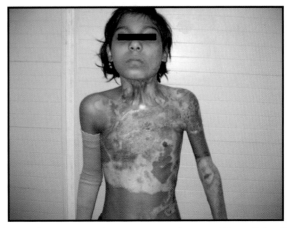

Fig. 5.13: Four weeks post-graft picture with well healed areas with start of hypertrophy of intergraft region

Two to four weeks: Epidermis is hyperplastic. New collagen bundles appear and older collagen disappears. Even the bed shows increased collagen formation.

Five to six weeks post-graft: Collagen deposition increase in graft and bed. Epidermis is hyperplastic with thin narrow rete pegs.

POSTOPERATIVE MANAGEMENT OF GRAFTED AREAS (FIGS 5.15A TO D)

- Mobilization should not be allowed for 2 weeks postgraft. Elastic support in the form of crepe bandage over a light dressing is given on extremities especially lower limbs to prevent venous congestion in grafts when weight bearing is started. This will prevent dehiscence of grafts.

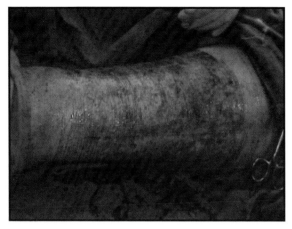

Fig. 5.14A: Thin split skin graft harvested from thigh. Donor site tends to bleed profusely after graft is harvested

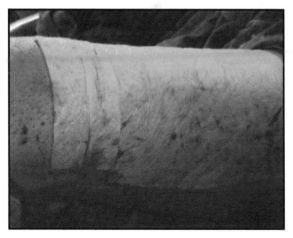

Fig. 5.14B: Donor area can also be dressed with dry collagen (skin temp)

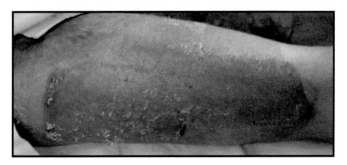

Fig. 5.14C: Typical appearance of same donor area after 10 days with hyperemia which disappears in the following days

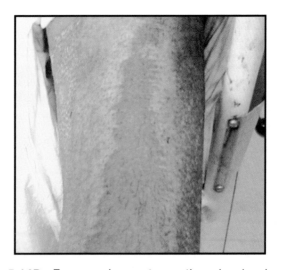

Fig. 5.14D: Four weeks postoperative showing hyperpigmentation with no scar hypertrophy as thin grafts were harvested

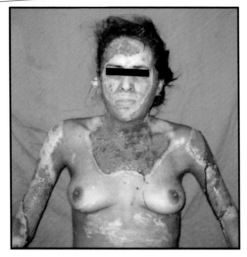

Fig. 5.15A: Post-burn raw area of face, neck, upper chest and upper arms, ready for grafting

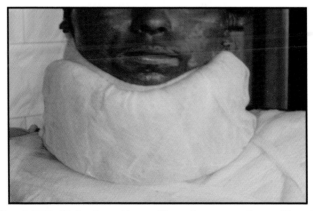

Fig. 5.15B: Following skin grafting of same patient with soft cervical collar to maintain position and prevent anterior contracture of neck. Collar has to be worn at all times except when exercising

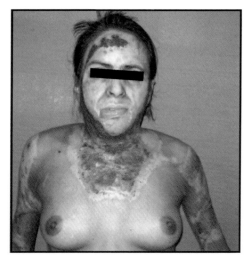

Fig. 5.15C: Late postoperative picture of same patient showing hyperpigmentation of grafts

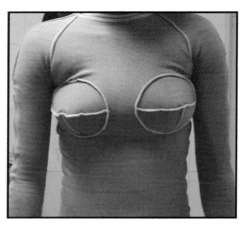

Fig. 5.15D: Customized pressure garments to be worn postoperative for at least 6 -12 months to provide pressure support to graft and help in its maturation

- At the same time measurements for pressure garments are taken and once the grafted area is fully healed and dry, the pressure garments are to be worn to provide pressure support for the graft. The importance of pressure garments can be explained by their following uses:

  1. They prevent venous congestion of graft and hemorrhagic blister formation.
  2. They prevent burning and tingling of limbs.
  3. Elevation of graft by underlying hematoma and rapid breakdown of newly epithelialized areas in early stages is also avoided.
  4. Helps in rapid maturation of graft and scar tissue making it more soft and pliable.
  5. In case of meshed grafts and where gaps are left in between two sheets of graft there can be hypertrophic scarring in the interstices. This causes a cobblestone appearance but this can be prevented by the pressure garments.

- Pressure garments have to be worn for 24 hours during the day and advised to be removed only for bathing, massaging or exercising. They have to be used for 12 - 18 months. Once the graft is completely mature these elastic supports can be removed.

- The grafted area shows drying and scaling and itching. This is because split skin grafts have no sweat or sebaceous glands so that they need to be kept lubricated with some oil.

- Hyperpigmentation of graft and donor areas is unpredictable but certain in patients with dark skin. Infact the shorter the distance between the donor and recipient sites the better the color match.

Hyperpigmentation can be minimized by avoiding exposure to sunlight and using sunscreen agents.

- Grafts take up sensory pattern of the recipient site because innervations of graft is from the deeper nerve branches and not from the margins. Return of the sensory pattern in grafted area is unpredictable.
- Splints have to be used for grafted areas over joints to minimize contracture formation.
- Physiotherapy has to be done to mobilize all parts of the body and return them to their original functional state and prevent deformities and functional restriction.

Biosynthetic Skin Substitutes

Are available as *Biobrane.* This is a bilaminar membrane of nylon mesh with a silicone sheet which adheres to the wound bed and promotes fibro vascular in growth. This is very expensive and has no added advantage over the other dressing materials. They are mainly used temporarily for covering excised wounds following full thickness burns or for coverage of superficial partial thickness burns.

Integra: It is another artificial skin available as a bilaminar membrane with collagen layer and silicone layer sheet which stimulates formation of neodermis over which split skin graft can be applied. Again this is very expensive. This is also usually used over raw areas following excision of wounds till such time that autografts can be applied.

Cultured Epidermal Autografts (CEA)

Involves tissue culture of epidermal cells from patients own skin which produces sheets of skin in 21 days which can be applied over raw area left after excising full thickness wounds. The disadvantage is the time taken to culture the skin. Another limiting factor is the expense of culturing tissue and nonavailability of the technique at all centers.

CHAPTER 6

General Treatment of Burn Patients

Emergency steps that have been discussed till now focus mainly on the resuscitation of the patient and treatment of associated injuries and emergency management of burn wound. Soon after the patient stabilizes and comes out of the acute phase, the focus shifts to general support of the patient which includes:

- Nutritional support
- General condition improvement
- Immunomodulatory support
- Pain management and psychosocial support
- Control of infection
- Rehabilitation.

IMPROVING GENERAL CONDITION

The overall general condition of the patient can be improved not only by improving nutrition of the patient but by maintaining the personal hygiene whish gives a feeling of well being to the patient. The patient should be given regular bath (Fig. 6.1) or shower which helps in removing all the loose debris and discharge without rubbing the wounds.

NUTRITION IN BURNS

Apart from infection, the hyper metabolic response to burn injury is the second most important factor affecting the morbidity and outcome for a burned patient. Any major burn disrupts the normal hormonal balance in the patient which can increase the BMR, oxygen consumption, increase nitrogen loss, increase lipolysis and therefore loss of body mass.

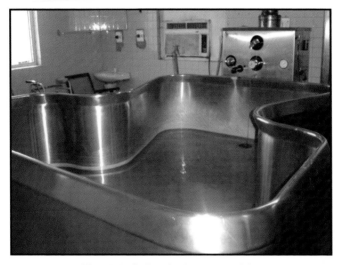

Fig. 6.1: Saline bath tub used for
giving bath to burn patient

Therefore, the main principle underlying successful treatment of a burn patient is in providing an adequate nutritional support.

Enteral nutrition is the method of choice. However, if the patient is not accepting well orally then total parental nutrition (TPN) should be administered. A nasogastric tube feeding can also be given to patients not taking adequate oral feeds. Burn patients are usually in a catabolic state till the wounds heal. Therefore, these patients normally require a high calorie and high protein diet in order to revert the negative nitrogen balance and prevent rapid weight loss. The patients with >25 percent burns cannot cope up with the caloric demands that the trauma imposes on them. These patients, therefore need enteral supplementation. About 50 percent calories should be supplied as carbohydrates, 20 percent as proteins and 30 percent of the calories should be supplied as fat. The ratio of calories to nitrogen in a hypercatabolic burn patient is approximately 135:1. At least 10 percent of the calories should be given as fat to prevent essential fatty acid deficiency. There are various formulae for the protein and caloric requirement.

Artz : Recommended 2 – 3 g protein /kg body wt + 50 – 70 g cal /kg body wt.

Sutherland : Gives the requirement in term of body weight and surface area burned.

In adults: Calories — 20 cal/kg wt + 70 cal/% BSA
Protein requirement — 1 g/kg wt + 3 g/% BSA

In children: Calorie requirement — 60 cal/kg wt + 35 cal/% BSA
Protein requirement – 3 g/kg wt +1 g/% BSA

Oral nutrition: The maximum amount that an adult can take orally is about 3000-4000 Kcal and 180 g proteins. For this burn patients need to take high calorie and high protein diet. There are readily available protein rich products which can be used.

Parenteral nutrition: In extensive burns IV supplements are to be given in the form of IV amino acids (e.g. hermin, alamin), fat (intralipid, lipofundin), 10 percent glucose and electrolytes and vitamins. Nowadays combined preparations are also available which give carbohydrates, fats and amino acids in a single pack like: Clinomel, Vitrimix. When such hyperosmolar solutions are used, CVP line is required for infusion to avoid thrombophlebitis.

When the patients wounds are almost covered, the diet should be gradually shifted from tube to IV feeds to oral feeds.

PREVENTION OF DEHYDRATION

Even after correction of shock in first two days after burns, there is danger of dehydration because of continuing evaporative losses from the wound surface. If not treated it can cause hypernatremia, weight loss, oliguria, raised serum osmolarity and septicemia. The evaporative losses have to be therefore calculated and corrected.

Evaporative water loss in ml / hr = (25+ BSA burn) × total body surface (m^2).

This amount has to be added to average daily requirements and insensible losses. As the wound start healing, the evaporative losses also decrease and therefore smaller volumes will be required.

ANEMIA

Apart from the red cell destruction in the acute burn, there is further loss of blood later on in the form of:

- Bleeding from raw area
- Hematemesis and melena
- Blood loss during dressing
- Operative blood loss
- Septicemia leading to hemolysis
- Hemoglobin estimation is therefore to be done weekly and is a fair indication for blood transfusion in order to raise Hb upto 100 percent.

ELECTROLYTE IMBALANCE

Is very common in burn patients.Most common being:

Hyponatremia: Because of overhydration especially in infants and children or in adults in whom only pure water is given in shock period.

Hypernatremia: When dehydration is allowed to prolong.

Hypokalemia: Occurs if losses of potassium in urine are more than intake though very small amount of potassium is lost from burn surface.

Hyperkalemia: In case of acute renal failure especially in electric burn.

These disturbances should be corrected before they cause irreversible damage.

CURLING'S ULCER PREVENTION

These stress ulcers are very common in burns patients. The best mode of prevention is enteral feeds which maintain gastric and intestinal mucosal integrity by ensuring the organ perfusion and providing material on which gastric acid can act. If the patient is not taking proper enteral feeds, they should be put on H_2 blockers and antacids.

DEEP VEIN THROMBOSIS PREVENTION (FIGS 6.2A AND B)

All burn patients are at risk of DVT if they are immobile. Therefore, early mobilization and ambulation are best prophylaxis for DVT along with low molecular weight heparin. Patients in ICU with extensive burns have to be specifically monitored for signs and symptoms of DVT and pulmonary embolism.

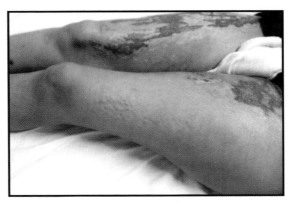

Fig. 6.2A: Deep vein thrombosis (DVT)of left lower leg in a patient suffering from 40 percent burns.Patient presented with severe pain in leg with increasing swelling of left thigh and leg and severe pain during movements of leg. Note the edematous left thigh compared to right thigh

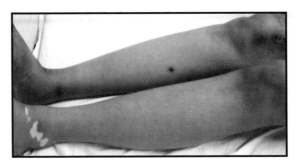

Fig. 6.2B: Same patient with swelling in left lower leg compared to right lower leg. Calf tenderness and Homan's sign positive in left leg indicating DVT. Color Doppler showed long thrombus in left external iliac and femoral vein

IMMUNOMODULATION

The first form of immunomodulation used in burns is *tetanus* prophylaxis by giving tetanus toxoid and tetanus immunoglobulin in case history of previous immunization is not available.

The second type of immunomodulation used in burn patients is in the form of *nutritional immunomodulators*, i.e. long chain fatty acids and amino acids. The potential role of certain amino acids particularly arginine and glutamine is still an area of active research. The role of glutamine which is the most common amino acid in the body has been studied extensively and is supposed to play an important role in hyper metabolic conditions like burns.

The third form of immunomodulation is by using specific *immunoglobulins* like Ig G (trade name –IV Glob) or Ig M or a combination of Ig G, A, M (trade name – pentaglobin). Pentaglobin is found to be very effective in improving the general condition if the patient goes into sepsis.

Pseudomonas immunoglobulin has been given prophylactically to major burn patients and has shown earlier return of immunoglobulin levels to normal and lower mortality.

Role of *steroids* is debatable. But in inhalational injury short-term steroids give good results because it decreases the inflammatory edema. But most surgeons believe that use of steroids have more disadvantages because it increases the patients susceptibility to infection and decreases wound healing.

CHAPTER 7

Systemic Antibiotics

Though antibiotics are widely used in burns, however, their use has always been controversial, since all the burn wounds are sterile to start with since all surface bacteria are killed by the heat. But because both cellular and humoral immunity is decreased in burns especially extensive burns, these patients are very susceptible to infection. In addition there is translocation of bacteria from the gut to the circulation if splanchnic vasoconstriction is prolonged. All these factors can be reduced by proper local wound management and proper fluid therapy. Prophylactic antibiotics do not decrease incidence of infection. Instead indiscriminate use of antibiotics can increase multiple resistant strains and also reduce the body's immune defence mechanism further. Thus it makes the patient more susceptible to invasive sepsis and makes the later on management of these patients a great challenge. Therefore, the use of *prophylactic antibiotics* is to be restricted to only a few cases which include:

- Markedly debilitated patient
- HIV positive patient
- Rheumatic heart disease
- Patient on pacemaker
- Patient with other implants in body
- Diabetes mellitus
- Antistreptococcal antibiotics can be given to infants and children for 24-48 hours when surgery or synthetic dressing is done as children are often colonized by these organisms and very sensitive to their growth.

Choice of Antibiotic

The best antibiotic which was earlier used for prophylaxis in burns was crystalline penicillin. The rationale behind using penicillin G in the first post-burn week, in the earlier days was to prevent group A –beta hemolytic streptococcal burn wound cellulitis and also the protection it gave the patient against infection by *Clostridium tetani*. Because even though Tetanus toxoid injection is routinely given to all patients, the action of TT comes only after 7-10 days. For this period when the patient is at risk of developing tetanus due to contaminated wounds and in the era when incidence of tetanus was high, Crystalline penicillin was given as a routine prophylaxis in all burns.

Regular wound culture and sensitivity is most essential to know how the wound colonizes and the best antibiotic to be used for the same. Antibiotics without culture sensitivity report are to be started only if signs and symptoms of systemic invasion or wound sepsis start appearing. Burn wound sepsis is suspected when colony count is $>10^5$org/g tissue.

Signs and Symptoms of Burn Wound Invasion (Figs 7.1 to 7.3)

- Black or dark brown focal areas of discoloration
- Satellite lesions
- Partial thickness wound converting to full thickness wound
- Increased pus discharge from wound because of sloughing of eschar or softening of eschar
- Discoloration of skin around the wound margins or surrounding cellulitis
- Hemorrhagic discoloration in subcutaneous tissue.

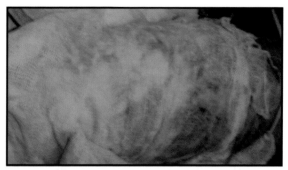

Fig. 7.1: Typical green discharge and discoloration of dressing indicating pseudomonas infection of wounds

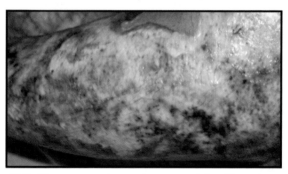

Fig. 7.2: Burn wound sepsis caused by *Pseudomonas aeruginosa* for the same patient as in Figure 7.1. Note the green staining of burn surface with focal areas of black discoloration

Signs and Symptoms of Systemic Septicemia (Figs 7.4 to 7.9)

When the organisms start invading the bloodstream are:
• Sudden rise or fall in temperature (<36.5° or >38.5°C) with rigors

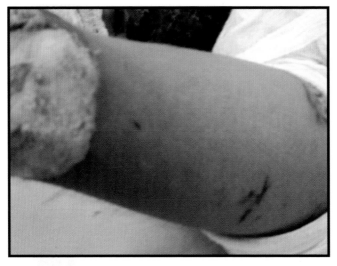

Fig. 7.3: Burn wound infection caused by streptococcus indicated by cellulitis in adjoining non burned areas

- Tachycardia
- Tachypnea (>40 breaths/min)
- Nausea and vomiting
- Diarrhea
- Hypotension
- Paralytic ileus
- Leukocytosis or leukopenia
- Altered mental status (confusion or delirium)
- Thrombocytopenia (< 50,000 platelets/mm^3).

Management of Burn Wound Sepsis

In these cases immediate debridement of infected eschar should be done to decrease bacterial load and change

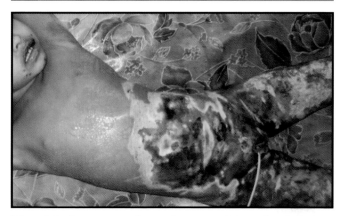

Fig. 7.4: Burn wound sepsis caused by mixed flora – Enterobacter and Klebsiella. The entire wound is converted into thick black eschar with systemic signs of sepsis

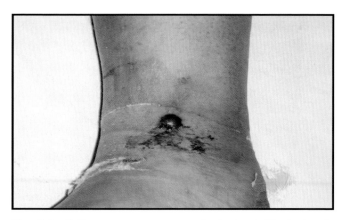

Fig. 7.5: Ecthyma gangrenosum –typical satellite lesion in gram-negative sepsis in the form of cutaneous vesicular lesion over normal uninvolved skin is a poor prognostic indicator

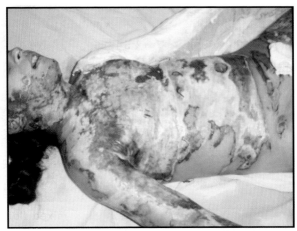

Fig. 7.6: Deep dermal burns converted to full thickness wounds due to pseudomonas infection

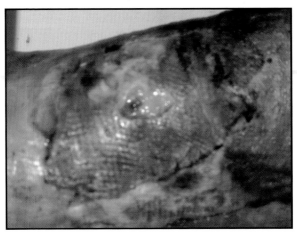

Fig. 7.7: Infection of grafted site with *Staphylococcus aureus*. Initial 'Take' of graft followed by typical eaten up appearance of graft. Immediate topical treatment with anti-staphylococcal ointments stopped the progression of destruction of the graft

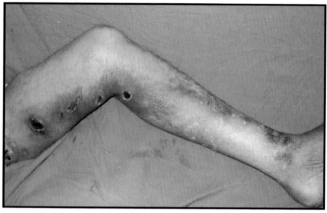

Fig. 7.8: Infective thrombophlebitis of entire lower leg along the path of great saphenous vein (GSV)due to infected IV site in lower leg.Patient had a IV cut down in GSV following which he developed fever, erythema of leg and satellite necrotic lesions all along the vein. Treatment was total excision of the GSV from site of infection to its entry into femoral vein

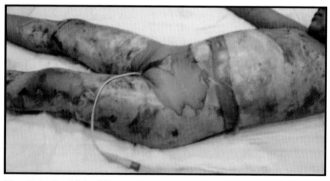

Fig. 7.9: A child with extensive scalds with burn wound sepsis. Partial thickness burns converting to full thickness burns with black areas of discoloration and increased pus discharge from the wounds

the topical antimicrobial agent. Mafenide has a greater role to play in burn wound sepsis because of its excellent penetration of burn eschar. A combination of broad spectrum antibiotics should be started as per the usual flora proliferating in the ward and their sensitivity pattern. Use of single antibiotic is to be avoided. Aminoglycoside dosage is to be individualized as per the patients renal condition.

Fungal infections are rarely seen in burn wounds but are difficult to diagnose and treat (Fig. 7.10). Most common fungal infection seen in burn patients is by Candida species

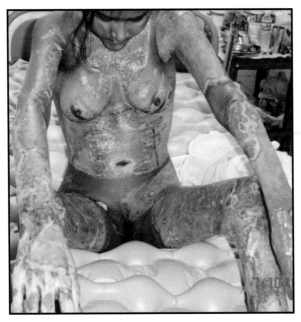

Fig. 7.10: Fungal infection of burn wounds
−3 weeks post-burn

and occurs two to three weeks post-burn. Is characterized by pain and itching in the wounds. This has to be treated with systemic antifungal agent like Amphotericin B and topical antifungal agents like mycostatin or nystatin powder.

Choice of Antibiotics for Burn Wound Sepsis

Organism	Antibiotics
Streptococcus	Penicillin group, macrolides (erythromycin)
Staphylococcus	Flucloxacillin, Cloxacillin, Methicillin, Vancomycin, Cephalosporins, Linezolid
Pseudomonas	Aminogycosides, Third generation cephalosporins, Piperacillin, Tazobactam/Sulbactam, Carbapenems (imipenem/meropenem)
Other gram-negative rods	Aminogycosides, Carbapenems (imipenem/meropenem)
MRSA (methicillin resistant *Staph aureus*)	Teicoplanin, Vancomycin, Lincomycin

CHAPTER 8

Inhalational Injury

Inhalational injury is very common in burn patients with an incidence of 33 percent in major burns. Its importance lies in the fact that it increases the mortality associated with burns.

Mode of Injury

1. *Thermal injury:* Because of direct effect of heat via the flames. Is usually restricted to area above vocal cords and results in mucosal blistering, ulceration and rapidly developing edema.

2. *Chemical injury:* Due to inhalation of smoke from burning toxic materials, fumes, mists and gases. These are more damaging than heat itself as toxic gases in the smoke and carbon particles along with other irritants coat the airway tract and these disrupt the epithelium, impair the mucociliary clearance and cause bronchoconstriction and increased mucus secretion.

3. *Systemic effects:* Are usually due to carbon monoxide and cyanide which are the two components of smoke. Carbon monoxide decreases the oxygen carrying capacity of hemoglobin because it has 200 times affinity for hemoglobin and it also prevents release of oxygen from oxyhemoglobin. Cyanide is released from burning plastic material and it causes tissue hypoxia by inactivating cytochrome oxidase and blocking oxygen utilization at cellular level.

Clinical Consequences of Inhalation Injury

- These patients are more hemodynamically unstable than patients with cutaneous burns only.

- Amount of fluid requirement during resuscitation is increased by 50 percent in these patients.
- Chances of pneumonia and ARDS increases chances of multiorgan failure.
- Injury to larynx and trachea can lead to voice impairment and subglottic stenosis.

Diagnosis

Is established by signs and symptoms.

History

- Mode of injury
- Exposure to smoke in closed spaces
- Duration of exposure.

Signs (Fig. 8.1)

- Black soot on face
- Black sputum
- Facial burns
- Singed nasal hair
- Hoarseness
- Tachypnea
- Stridor
- Respiratory distress.

Signs of Carbon Monoxide and Cyanide Toxicity

- Headache
- Altered mental status

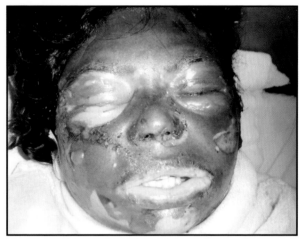

Fig. 8.1: Flame injuries to face due to bursting of kerosene oil stove causing severe soft tissue edema of face including eyelids and lips with singeing of nasal hair –all indicators of inhalational injury

- Dyspnea
- Weakness
- Tachycardia
- CO toxicity specifically shows normal PaO_2 and O_2 saturation on ABG and pulse oximetry and increased carboxyhemoglobin levels
- In cyanide toxicity there is odour of bitter almonds and high anion gap metabolic acidosis despite oxygen therapy and adequate fluid resuscitation.

Investigations

- Pulse oximeter gives continous measurement of oxygenation which is dependent on perfusion.

- ABG gives more definitive assessment of pulmonary gas exchange. Early hypoxia indicates severe injury. Initial ABG report gives a baseline for comparison in later stages as lung function worsens.
- Carbon monoxide toxicity is established by measuring COHb levels (< 15% are toxic and > 50% are lethal).
- Persistent metabolic acidosis indicates cyanide toxicity.
- Cyanide levels > 0.5 microgm/ml are potentially toxic and > 3 microgm/ml are lethal.
- Chest X-ray is normal in early stages.
- *Fiberoptic bronchoscopy:* It is the best mode and gives detail picture of supraglottic structures and tracheobronchial tract. The presence of infraglottic soot and inflammatory changes suggest inhalation injury.
- IV Xenon-133 ventilation perfusion scanning helps in identifying small airway obstruction following inhalation injury as these areas retain isotope for >90 sec.

Guidelines for Management

- Inhalation injury increases volume of fluid required for resuscitation.
- Inhalation injury increases the risk of ARDS and other pulmonary complications with severe cutaneous burns. Therefore specific supportive treatment for airway and breathing is a priority.
- Airway edema and occlusion develop rapidly so early endotracheal intubation is indicated prophylactically if the patient is hypoxic, mental status is depressed with deep burns to head and neck or other signs and symptoms of airway obstruction.

- Standard treatment for patient with carbon monoxide toxicity is 100 percent oxygen by mask or endotracheal tube(Fig. 8.3).
- In case cyanide toxicity is suspected, treatment is started empirically by giving Sodium thiosulphate 150 mg/kg over 15 min. This converts cyanide to thiocyanate, which is nontoxic.
- In circumferential full thickness burns the chest wall compliance is decreased and ventilation impaired. In these cases, escharotomies are performed in anterior axillary line and are connected to transverse subcostal incision (Fig. 8.2).
- In case the escharotomy does not give relief and endotracheal intubation is difficult, urgent tracheostomy is indicated to deliver humidified oxygen (Fig. 8.6).

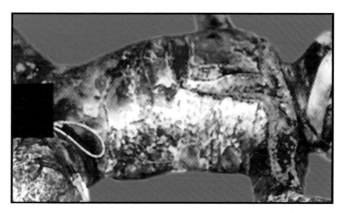

Fig. 8.2: Escharotomy incision in chest in case of full thickness burns of chest causing respiratory distress

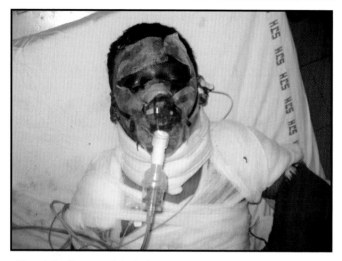

Fig. 8.3: Oxygen inhalation by mask in 25 percent burns with inhalation injury

- For majority of the patients, intubation is required only for a short duration till the upper airway edema subsides.
- Respiratory care requires airway suctioning and therapeutic bronchial lavage for removal of retained secretions and fibrin casts which cannot be cleared by the patient himself because of impaired mucociliary apparatus and ineffective coughing.
- Chest physiotherapy, postural drainage with head end elevation and coughing and early ambulation are also useful to improve lung function.
- Bronchodilators are useful for patients with bronchospasm especially in patients with a pre-existing reactive airway disease.

- Aerosolized adrenaline is used as a vasoconstrictor to reduce airway mucosal and sub-mucosal vascular congestion and edema.
- Role of steroids is controversial. Some centers use it on a short-term basis to reduce edema because of anti-inflammatory action. Others associate their use with a greater risk of infection.
- Mechanical ventilation is required in patients with moderate to severe inhalational injury in order to prevent respiratory failure (Figs 8.4 and 8.5).

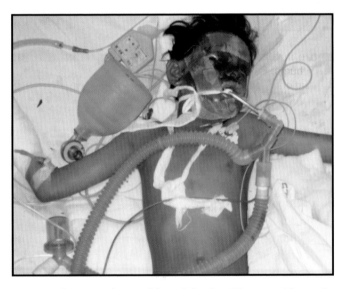

Fig. 8.4: Severe edema of face following 20 percent burns in a child. Management of airway with early intubation. Patient could be extubated after 72 hours following decrease in tissue edema

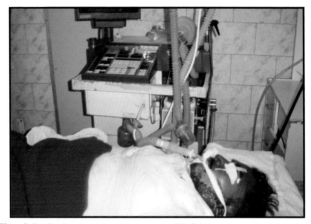

Fig. 8.5: Patient with 65 percent TBSA burns with history of smoke inhalation due to fire in a closed space, without any facial burns. Patient required intubation and was on mechanical ventilation

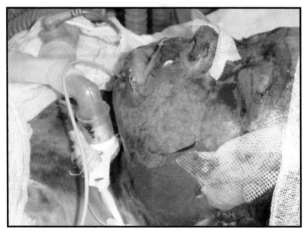

Fig. 8.6: Severe full thickness burns of face, neck and chest. Endotracheal intubation was difficult honoo trachostomy was mandatory in this case

- There are various modes used for ventilation but usually (a) volume assisted control mode or (b) SIMV (synchronized intermittent mandatory ventilation. Or (c) high frequency percussive ventilation mode (HFPV) is used for these patients.
- Mechanical ventilation is withdrawn as soon as edema subsides and patient starts maintaining SPO_2 on spontaneous ventilation.
- Prophylactic antibiotic have to be started early as respiratory tract infection is the most common complication following inhalational injury.

CHAPTER 9

Electrical Burns

Factors which affect severity of electric burns are:
- Amperage
- Voltage
- Alternating or direct current
- Frequency
- Duration of contact
- Path of current through body
- Resistance of skin or body parts

Causes of death from electric burn are:
- Respiratory failure
- Ventricular fibrillation - most common cause

CLASSIFICATION OF ELECTRICAL BURNS

1. *High voltage burns* (Fig. 9.1) by contact with high voltage electric lines ranging from 10,000 to 32,000 volts. The tissues are so extensively and rapidly damaged that they usually involve amputation of a

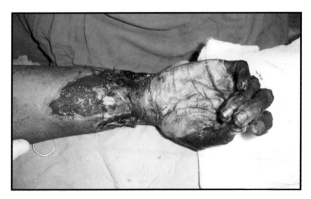

Fig. 9.1: Deep burns to hand and wrist by contact with high voltage lines producing claw deformity by spastic contracture of flexor muscles and gangrene of all fingers

limb either partly or completely. In these cases the damage actually extends into the normal tissues quite proximal to the apparently affected areas. This is to be kept on mind while doing amputation as the level of amputation can be higher than what is planned because of proximally damaged muscles below the normal skin.

2. *Low voltage electrical burns* (Figs 9.2A and B) are caused by low voltage (240 AC) domestic appliances. Though more common than the high voltage burns they may be deceptive in appearance as they may penetrate deeply. They are very commonly seen in infants crawling on the floor or in children who take the electrical wires into their mouth and chew them (Figs 9.3A and B). They suffer severe damage to the lips, tongue and mouth and though the legion may be small the reactive edema may interfere with breathing and may require tracheostomy.

3. *Electrothermal burns*: Results from accidental contact with elements of electrical instruments. Especially seen amongst children.

4. *Electrical flash burns* (Figs 9.4 and 9.5): Results from fire resulting from electrical sparks or flash. Degree of damage depends upon the time duration of exposure to the flash or the proximity of the patient to the actual flash.

5. *Electric shock:* Results from current passing through the entire body. It usually does not produce cutaneous burns but has more severe affects on central nervous system, cardiovascular system and other systems of the body. The patient usually suffers from trembling,

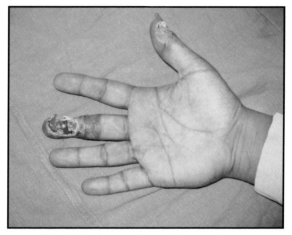

Fig. 9.2A: Low voltage injury to fingers leading to exposed tendons and joint

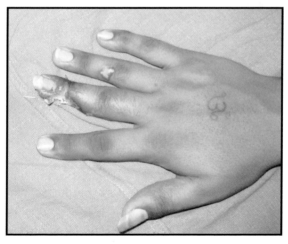

Fig. 9.2B: Dorsal aspect of hand of same patient

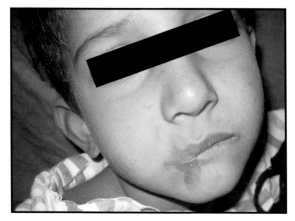

Fig. 9.3A: Post-burn scarring following low voltage injury by child chewing on electric wire

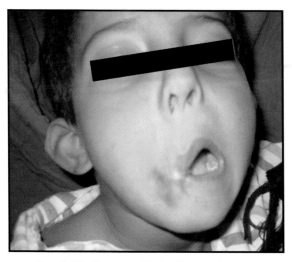

Fig. 9.3B: Same patient with mouth open showing ocverity of microstomia

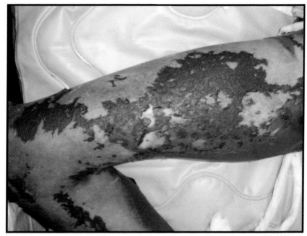

Fig. 9.4: Electric flash burns producing superficial burns in thigh and leg

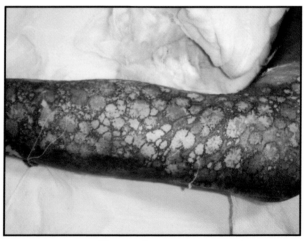

Fig. 9.5: Electric flash burns producing superficial dermal burns

sweating, pallor. Intracranial pressure may be raised and patient may become unconscious because of cerebral edema. There may be temporary deafness, auditory hallucinations, paralysis, stiffness of limbs, sudden blindness from retinal detachment or cataract at a later stage. Delayed neurological affects are rare. Apnea or cardiac arrest is the most severe presentation which requires immediate manual cardiopulmonary resusitaton (CPR).

6. *Lightening injuries* have variable affects. It may not always be fatal but patient may fall unconscious and stop breathing. However, these patient withstand prolong periods of apnea and respond very well to immediate CPR. Burn markings are characteristic for lightening injuries. There is a spidery pattern of skin burns which is caused by the currents passage along pathway of skin dampness where the resistance is the lowest.

Pathophysiology of Electric Burns

To understand the electrical burn injury, one must remember that like thermal burns where the injury is directly proportional to the amount of heat, in electrical injuries the damage is directly proportional to the electrical current which has flown into the body which inturn depends upon the voltage and the time that the electric current has flown in. However, in the electrical current, another factor comes in, that is the tissue resistance, less current flows but at that point electrical current is converted into heat energy and more heat destruction is seen. In this regard conventionally we say that this depends upon the laws of movement of electric current that is Ohm's law according to which I = V/R that is current is directly proportional to voltage and inversely proportional to resistance. Similarly heat production is directly dependent upon the Joule's law which states that heat is equal to 0.24 V^2 multiplied by resistance. These two simple laws explain about the movement of electrical current and the generation of heat. It is believed that various tissues offer different resistance and therefore at different places varying flow of current and generation of heat must be expected.

The affect of electrical burns depends upon the local damage as well as the systemic affect of the current. The local affect depends upon the place of contact, duration of contact and the voltage of current. Drier the skin, more local damage will be there and if the flexor surfaces have come in contact with the current, severe spasm of flexor muscles leads to tight holding of the wires and therefore prolonged contact and more damage. Severe spasms of flexor muscle may sometimes lead to fractures while similar injury where extensor surfaces have come in contact leads to spasm of extensor muscles and opisthotonus position and the patient is thrown away from the wire. Thus in such cases there is minimal amount of current flow and thus minimal local and systemic effects. In the tissues where there is least amount of conductivity, more local damage is seen like in the hand where there is massive damage to the skin because of excessive heat generation. After damage to the skin, the wet surface of the tendons, interosseii and lumbricals allows the current to flow. Then the current flows towards the wrist, the vessels supplying the skin are destroyed by the movement of the current and this leads to total avascular necrosis of the skin around the wrist on the volar aspect. On the dorsal aspect, at most places the blood supply is from the perforating branches coming from different muscles, in addition to direct branches coming from carpal and metacarpal vascular network. Therefore less local damage is seen on the dorsal aspect. Similarly when the current flows upward with the good flexor muscle mass and good perforating network of vessels supplying the volar aspect of forearm, no further damage to the skin is noticed. By the time, current reaches the elbow there is very little muscle mass, and the current comes in contact with the skin leading to further heat damage to the skin because of increased resistance of the skin. Similar effect is seen when the current flows upward throw the thick muscle mass of the arms, but by the time it reaches near the axilla on the medial side, muscle mass reduces and current comes in contact with the skin of higher resistance leading to damage of skin in axilla. This preferential damage has been explained as the "arcing" phenomenon (Fig. 9.6). Though there is no arcing or jumping of current anywhere in the body.

Electric burn wounds: Are variable and depend upon the type of electric burn. For contact burns, the usual entry point (Figs 9.7 and 9.8) is charred and depressed and swelling extends proximal from entry wound indicating the damage to underlying tissues by heat generated by the passage of current. The exit wound (Fig. 9.9) appears as though the current has exploded out of the skin with dry, depressed margins. The skin lesions may vary from small spots which are ischemic, yellowish white to larger

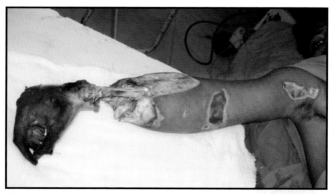

Fig. 9.6: High voltage electric injury causing complete destruction of wrist and arc phenomenon in elbow and axilla. The hand is totally devascularized

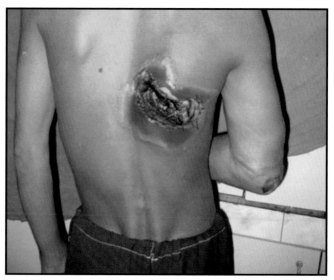

Fig. 9.7: Entry wound of electric burn due to contact with high tension wires

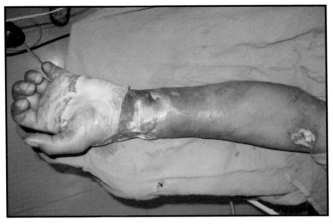

Fig. 9.8: Entry wound in hand from contact with high tension wire

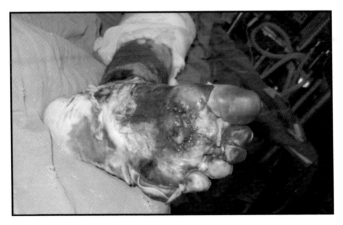

Fig. 9.9: Exit wound in the foot of the same patient as shown in Figure 9.8 as patient was standing on the ground

areas of charring. Necrosis of tissue is the main feature and may extend to tissues depeer than the skin. A limb may seem viable initially but may become ischemic and gangrenous later on because the damage in deeper tissues is always progressive in electric burns. Since the current flows through blood vessels which are good conductors there is a greater damage to the venous system as compared to the arterial system because in veins the per unit of current is higher because of slow movement of current. Whereas in arteries because of rapid flow of current the per unit of current changes very rapidly. However, the early venous damage in the form of venous thrombosis eventually leads to retrograde arterial thrombosis (Fig. 9.10). Therefore what previously appeared as live tissue becomes dead because of this

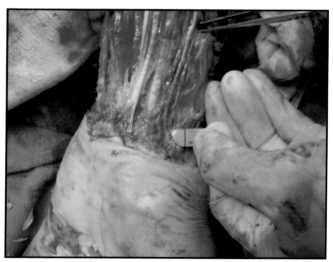

Fig. 9.10: Early debridement of full thickness burns following electric contact burns showing thrombosed veins

subsequent arterial thrombosis. This explains the progressive nature of damage associated with high voltage electrical burns.

In arc burns the burns are also severe and deep. Flash burns caused by ignition of clothing by electrical sparks are usually superficial to deep like usual thermal burns depending on time of contact.

MANAGEMENT

- The first and foremost reaction in case of electric injury is to immediately switch off the current supply and to remove the victim from the source of electric current with the help of some insulated material or wooden object in case the current is not cut off so as to avoid electrocution of the rescuer himself.
- If the patient is not breathing or heart is not beating, CPR is to be started and continued till the patient can be moved to the hospital.
- *Fluid resuscitation:* For low voltage burns, hardly any fluid replacement is required. However, in high voltage injuries in which apart from rapid loss of fluid into the areas of damage, there is also release of myoglobin from the dead muscles into the circulation. For this reason, this is considered very similar to a crush injury and require larger amounts of fluid replacement. Fluid requirement cannot be calculated as per the percentage of BSA as that may be small, yet the actual damage to underlying tissue and muscle may be more extensive. Therefore, the fluids in the form of ringer lactate is to be infused rapidly to produce a good urine output and the aim has to be to keep output at about 2 ml/

kg/hr for first 48 hours. CVP monitoring can help in preventing fluid overload.

- Reddish black urine color indicates hemoglobinuria and myoglobinuria because of hemolysis and muscle damage. These pigments can cause distal tubular necrosis and blockage of tubules leading to acute renal failure. This can be prevented by copious amount of IV fluids and by giving IV mannitol (1 ml/kg).

- In addition to this, the urine is to be made alkaline by giving IV sodabicarbonate (50 cc 8 hourly) Check the urine pH–if still acidic, increase the dose of sodabicarbonate.

- In case of flash burns, the fluid replacement is principally the same as in thermal burns.

- Apart from tetanus toxoid, in case of high voltage injury where there is gangrenous changes, prophylactic dose of human tetanus immunoglobulin (TIG) should also be administered in a dose of 250-500 IU intramuscularly. In rare case which come late with features of tetanus setting in, therapeutic dose of TIG should be given, i.e. 3000-6000 IU in divided doses (though some believe that a single dose of 500 IU also suffices).

Wound Management

- For small burns as in low voltage injuries or flash burns the area is to be treated like any thermal burns with local anti-microbial creams and allowed to heal. Or small areas can even be taken up for excision and grafting. In case the neurovascular bundles or joints are exposed local flaps are used for covering to protect the underlined structures from further damage (Figs 9.11A and B).

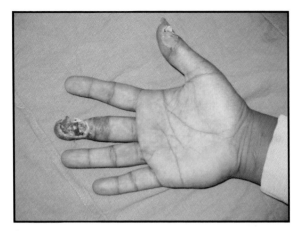

Fig. 9.11A: Low voltage injury to finger with exposed tendon and bone

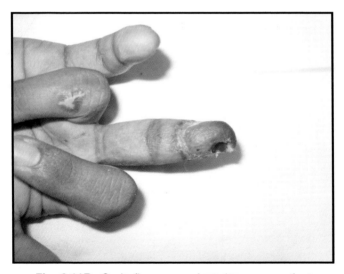

Fig. 9.11B: Groin flap cover given for same patient

- In high voltage injuries, involving the extremities, relaxing incisions in the eschar (escharotomy) or even a fasciotomy is indicated so that the edema under the tight dry eshcar may not compromise the blood supply of the limb (Figs 9.12 to 9.14).
- In case dead muscles are seen in the incision lines after the patient's general condition stabilizes, the patient is to be taken up for debridement and dressing. It may be necessary to do serial debridement in order to remove all the dead tissues as damage is progressive in electrical injury. This is to be followed by either a split skin grafting or a flap cover (Figs 9.15A and B). The aim is to protect the life of the patient by removing all the dead muscles.
- In case of very severe damage where the extremity shows frank gangrene,amputation is advisable as soon as line of demarcation sets in. Infact initially only a guillotine amputation is done and stump left open. This can be followed by a proper revised amputation as it frequently becomes necessary to amputate a few inches higher (Figs 9.16 and 9.17).
- In case of gangrene of upper limb, if amputation is required at shoulder level, there are chances of blow out from the stump of axillary vessels later on, which can be very difficult to control. To avoid this, the subclavian vessels are ligated by a supraclavicular approach (Figs 9.18A to D).
- In case entry and exit wounds are involving the chest or abdomen, intra-abdominal involvement is to be ruled out. For this chest X-ray and X-ray abdomen may be done as baseline investigation. Patient may

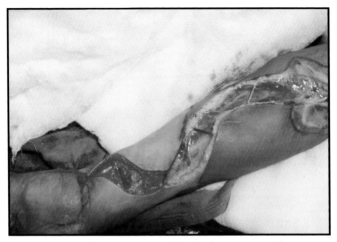

Fig. 9.12: Fasciotomy incision in forearm to release increased compartment pressure due to high voltage injury

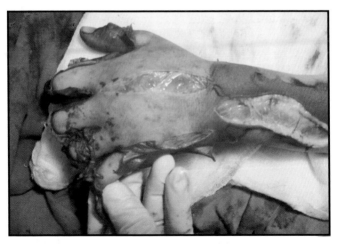

Fig. 9.13: Escharotomy incision on dorsum of hand

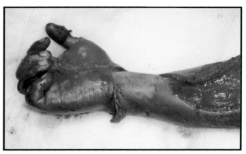

Fig. 9.14: Forearm incisions extending
into palm to open up carpal tunnel

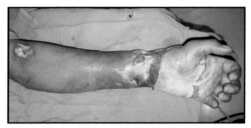

Fig. 9.15A: Full thickness burns over wrist because of
contact with high tension wire

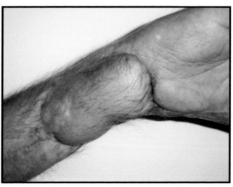

Fig. 9.15B: Debridement in same case with groin flap covers
over wrist to protect exposed tendons and neurovascular
bundles

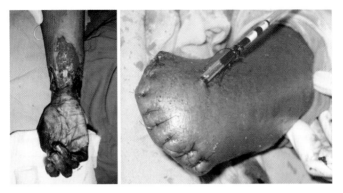

Fig. 9.16: Amputation stump following below elbow amputation for gangrene of hand and forearm following electric burn

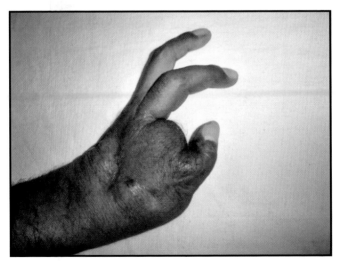

Fig. 9.17: Amputated index finger with groin flap cover over exposed metacarpal and first web space following electric contact burns

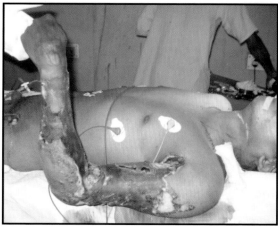

Fig. 9.18A: High voltage electric contact burn of both upper arms requiring bilateral shoulder amputation. A chance of blow out of axillary vessels is high following amputation

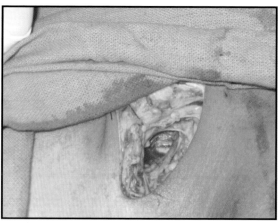

Fig. 9.18B: Same patient requiring ligation of subclavian vessels prior to shoulder amputation to avoid blow out distally. Supraclavicular approach used to expose subclavian vessels. Clavicle may be divided also if exposure is limited

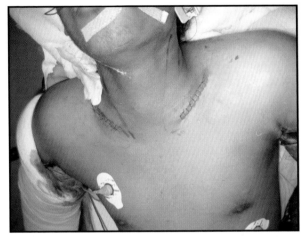

Fig. 9.18C: Bilateral subclavian vessels ligated through supraclavicular approach in same patient

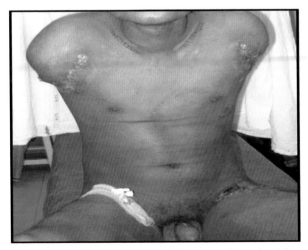

Fig. 9.18D: Postoperative picture of same patient after bilateral shoulder disarticulation and subclavian vessel ligation

be kept nil orally with Ryle's tube aspiration till intra-abdominal injury is completely ruled out. If depth of damage is superficial, only dressings are required and raw areas are grafted later.

- If there is abdominal wall rupture (Fig. 9.19), action needs to be taken fast or else the outcome is always fatal. The bowel injury has to be looked into by the general surgeons and the defect in the wall is to be reconstructed by some local flaps. Usually groin flap or tensor fascia lata flap or rectus abdominis flap is used depending upon the site of defect.

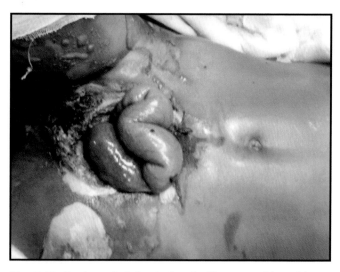

Fig. 9.19: Rupture of abdominal wall with exposed bowel loops following accidental fall of high voltage wires on the abdomen. Such patients have a high mortality if treatment is delayed

Following debridement major vessels may be left exposed many times. This is a problem which if neglected initially may present in a dramatic manner later on. Since blood vessels are good conductors, their walls are partly damaged though continuity is maintained. These partly damaged vessel walls can be salvaged if further anoxic damage is prevented. Bleeding from blowout of a major vessel can cause rapid exsanguination and death. In case bleeding vessel is ligated, the distal part of limb will be threatened. So to prevent this complication it is important to give primary cover to exposed vessels between 3rd-5th day. Wherever possible muscle or musculocutaneous flaps are preferred. A vascularized flap provides a capillary network to nourish the vessel wall and protect it from further damage (Figs 9.20A to 9.24D).

Areas where major vessels are exposed	Flaps used
Wrist	Groin flap
	Hypogastric flap
	Abdominal flap
Elbow	Latissimus dorsi flap
	Radial forearm flap
	Abdominal flap
Axilla	Pectoralis major flap
	Latissimus dorsi flap
Femoral triangle	Gracilis flap
	Rectus abdominis flap
Popliteal fossa	Gastrocnemius flap
	Free latissimus dorsi flap

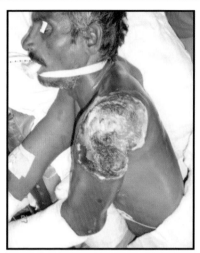

Fig. 9.20A: High tension contact burn over shoulder exposing joint and dead necrotic muscles

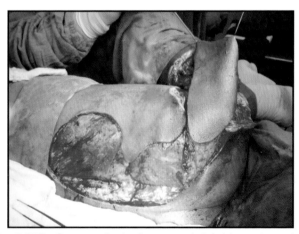

Fig. 9.20B: Same patient after wound debridement required a flap cover for which Trapezius musculocutaneous flap was raised

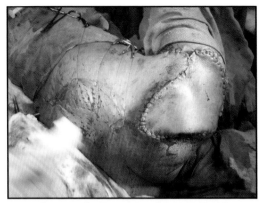

Fig. 9.20C: Trapezius flap inset with skin graft over donor site

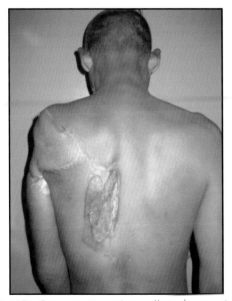

Fig. 9.20D: One month postoperative picture of same patient in posterior view

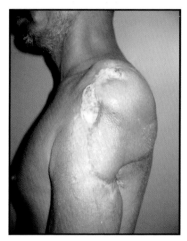

Fig. 9.20E: Lateral view of same patient

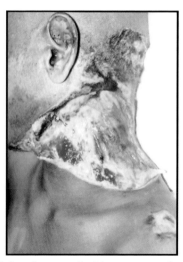

Fig. 9.21A: High voltage contact burns on neck exposing dead muscles with risk of blow out of carotid vessels if left as such

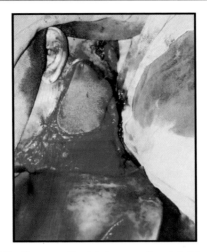

Fig. 9.21B: Same patient taken up for debridement and
ipsilateral pectoralis major flap cover

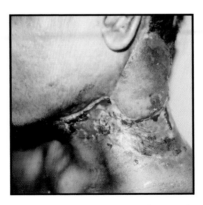

Fig. 9.21C: Two weeks postoperative picture showing healthy
muscle and skin paddle over it which avoided a catastrophe
of a major vessel blow out

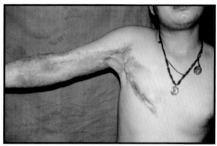

Fig. 9.22A: Another patient in whom an ipsilateral pectoralis major flap was used to cover exposed axillary vessels following electrical burns

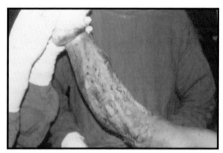

Fig. 9.22B: Latissimus dorsi flap for cover of brachial vessels at elbow following debridement of electrical burn wound

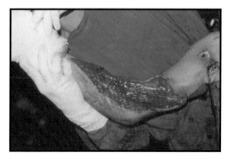

Fig. 9.22C: Same flap as in Figure 9.22B with graft applied over the flap

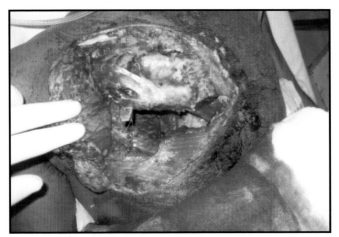

Fig. 9.23A: High voltage contact burns to right side of chest exposing ribs and lungs

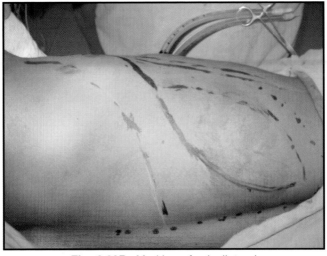

Fig. 9.23B: Markings for ipsilateral musculocutaneous latissimus dorsi flap

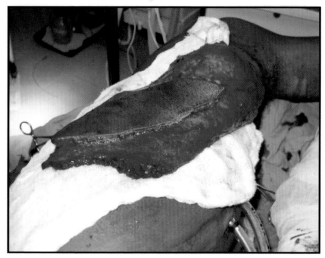

Fig. 9.23C: Raised musculocutaneous
latissimus dorsi (LD) flap

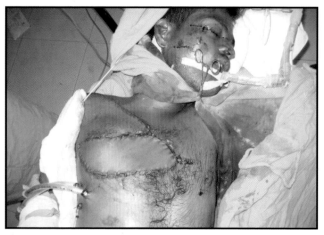

Fig. 9.23D: Inset LD flap for same patient with chest tube
drainage for re-expanding the lung

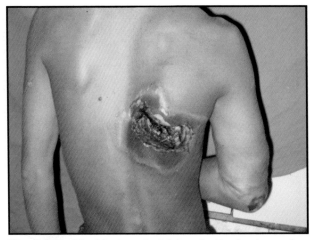

Fig. 9.24A: Electrical contact injury to the back causing exposure of ribs

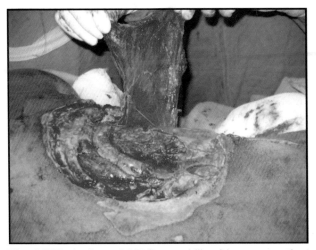

Fig. 9.24B: Ipsilateral LD flap mobilized in same patient following debridement

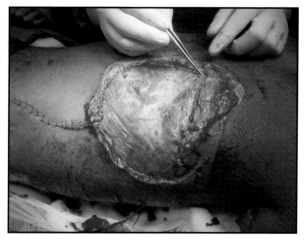

Fig. 9.24C: Transposed LD flap to cover ribs and renal angle area

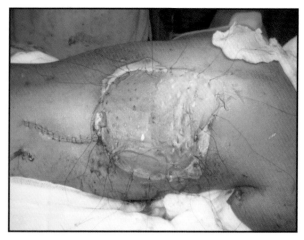

Fig. 9.24D: LD flap covered with skin graft over which tie over dressing was applied

- In case entry point is in the scalp, the damage is quite severe leading to involvement of skull bones. Depending on depth of damage, only bones may be exposed or dura may also be exposed. These cases have to be taken up for early debridement and cover as soon as the patients general condition stabilizes. If only bone is exposed, local scalp rotation or transposition flaps may be done or distant flap like radial forearm flap can be used. If dura or brain is exposed, bony cover under the skin flap will be required. Usually split rib graft or cranial bone grafts are used (Figs 9.25A to 9.26B).
- In majority of the high voltage injuries, there is often a history of fall from height. Therefore, associated head injury and spinal injury is to be ruled out early. For this, X-ray skull, X-ray cervicothoracic spine, CT scan head are very important. In case of head injury, neurosurgical intervention may be required. In spinal injury, conservative management is essential and supportive treatment for paraplegia or quadriplegia will be required.

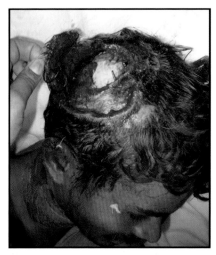

Fig. 9.25A: Full thickness burns to scalp and skull following contact with high tension wires. Patient also developed brain abscess

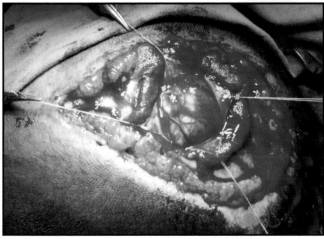

Fig. 9.25B: Same patient with craniectomy to remove dead bone and exposure of meninges

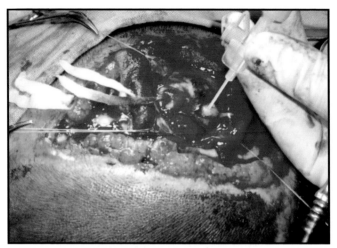

Fig. 9.25C: Abscess being drained in same patient

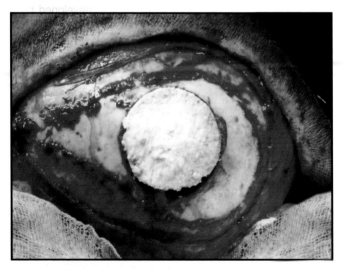

Fig. 9.25D: Covering bone defects with cranial bone graft

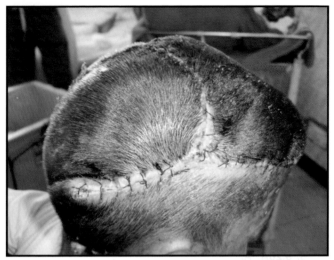

Fig. 9.25E: Transposition flap from adjoining normal scalp to cover the defect in the same patient

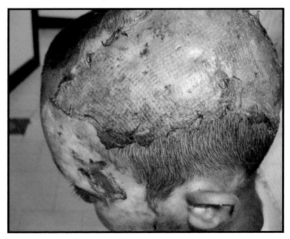

Fig. 9.25F: Donor area covered with split skin graft

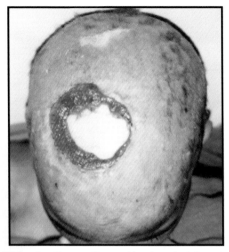

Fig. 9.26A: Another patient with electric injury to scalp. Only outer table was involved and inner table was healthy

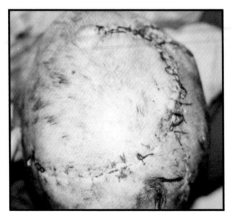

Fig. 9.26B: Rotation flaps to cover the defect in the scalp in the same patient

CHAPTER 10

Chemical Burns

Chemical burns are usually seen in the following settings:
1. Laboratory accidents—usually acids and alkalis
2. Domestic accidents—drain cleaners, toilet cleaners which contain acids or alkalis or paint removers, bleaching agents or deodorants and sanitizers (phenol).
3. Industrial accidents—acids, lye, inorganic compounds, molten metals, hot molten materials.
4. Medical accidents—potassium permanganate, dimethylsulfoxide.

Chemical burns can also be homicidal. In these cases usually the face, hands and chest are involved.

CLASSIFICATION OF CHEMICALS

According to Composition

1. *Acids*
    — sulphuric acid
    — hydrochloric acid
    — hydrofluoric acid
    — nitric acid
    — chromic acid
2. *Alkalis*
    — lime
    — caustic soda
    — caustic potash
    — ammonia
3. *Inorganic compounds*
    — phosphorus
    — sodium
    — cyanide
    — carbide
    — magnesium
    — cement

4. *Organic compounds*
   — cresol
   — lysol
   — phenol
   — methyl bromide
   — kerosene oil
   — petrol

According to Mechanism of Action

1. *Oxidizing agents*
   — chromic acid
   — potassium permanganate
   — sodium hypochlorite
   — nitric acid
2. *Corrosives*
   — phenols
   — white phosphorus
   — lyes (alkalis)—KOH, Na OH, NH$_4$ OH, LiOH, Ca(OH)$_3$, Ba$_2$ (OH)$_3$
   — lime
3. *Protoplasmic poisons*—strong acids
   — tungstic acid
   — picric acid
   — tannic acid
   — trichloroacetic acid
   — formic acid
   — cresylic acid
4. *Dessicants*
   — sulphuric acid
   — muriatic acid
5. *Vessicants*
   — cantharides
   — DMSO

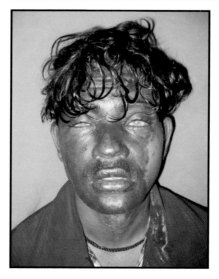

Fig. 10.1: Acid burns to face causing superficial burns

MECHANISM OF ACTION

Local Effects

Acids (Fig. 10.1) damage skin and tissues by:

a. Their hydrogen ions which breach the protective keratin layer of skin and causes coagulative necrosis of proteins.

b. Hygroscopic action –because of their affinity for water leading to desiccation of tissues.

c. Precipitation of proteins leads to exothermic reaction– heat liberated causes further thermal damage.

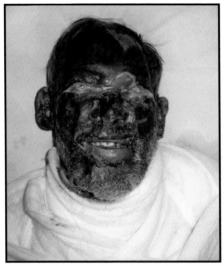

Fig. 10.2: Alkali burns causing deep full thickness injury to face and neck, involving both eyes—homicidal case

Alkalis (Fig. 10.2)– Act through
a. Hydroxyl ion by forming alkali proteinates which are soluble and therefore,the hydroxyl ion passes deeper into the cell and then from one cell to another thus penetrating deeper into the skin.
b. Saponification of fats by liquefaction process thus penetrating deep into the subcutaneous tissue. Hence the extent of damage is more extensive in case of alkali burns compared to acid burns.
c. Hygroscopic action which desiccates tissue.
d. Lime (Calcium oxide) in presence of water forms calcium hydroxide with production of heat because it involves an exothermic reaction.

Systemic Effects

Are seen in some chemicals especially organic compounds which get absorbed quickly from skin or by inhalation and effect the different organs. Like phenol gets absorbed from skin and leads to renal failure. Heavy metal poisoning occurs by absorption of organic metal complexes.

Factors affecting damage by chemicals:

1. Concentration of chemical
2. Duration of contact
3. Quantity of chemical
4. Mechanism of action
5. How early treatment is started.

Usually the amount of damage in chemical burns is more extensive than thermal burns because the chemical agent causes progressive damage till it gets inactivated by tissue reaction.

GENERAL PRINCIPLES OF MANAGEMENT

Most important aspect of treatment for chemical burns is the speed of treatment.

- Garments have to be removed quickly.
- Litmus test is done to ascertain whether agent is an acid or alkali if history is not known (Fig. 10.3).
- Excepting a few chemical agents, in most of the chemical injuries, the affected areas have to be copiously irrigated with water till litmus test is negative.
- If possible, showers should be used to wash off the chemicals (Fig. 10.4). This water dilution decreases the rate of reaction between the chemical and the tissue and also restores the pH of the affected area.

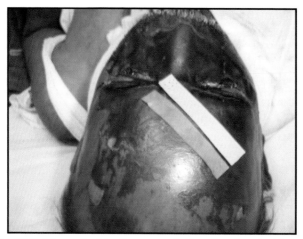

Fig. 10.3: Litmus test to diagnose whether the chemical is acid or alkali and also to check whether chemical has been completely washed off the wounds or not. Blue litmus paper changing to pink indicates acid present in wounds. Pink litmus paper changing to blue indicates alkali burn

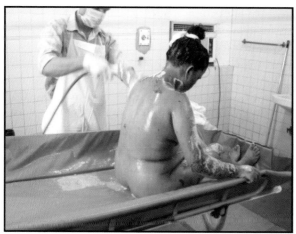

Fig. 10.4: Shower given to wash off the chemical

- Time should not be wasted in searching for specific antidotes. Infact the use of a neutralizing agent may produce heat by the exothermic reaction which can cause further tissue damage.
- There are certain agents in which use of water is contraindicated like sodium.
- For corneal burns, it is most important to wash with water continuously for atleast 30 min in order to avoid corneal damage which is irreversible.
- Water irrigation is usually indicated for 2 hours in acid burns and 12 hours in alkali burns.
- Patient should be immediately transferred to a burn unit taking care to continue irrigation during transfer as well.
- If a large area is involved, the other general principles for resuscitation are the same as for thermal burns.
- The specific treatment required for certain compounds is described later.
- If there are symptoms of systemic toxicity, they have to be dealt with accordingly.
- In case of accidental ingestion of corrosives there is a strong likelihood of *esophageal injury* especially if there are signs of corrosive injury in the posterior tongue and hypopharynx. After the general initial management, diagnostic esophagoscopy is to be done to see the extent of injury. There is a risk of iatrogenic esophageal perforation during this procedure especially if the esophagoscope is passed through areas of deep burns. So this should be avoided especially in case there is history of ingestion of alkalis as the depth of damage is greater in case of alkalis making the chances

of perforation higher, thus increasing the mortality. Whereas, in case of acid ingestion since depth of damage is less and survival chances are better, hence chances of stricture formation are more later on. In case of ingestion of caustics, esophageal fluoroscopy with a water soluble contrast material can show features of injury to the esophageal mucosa.

There are different approaches for treatment of esophageal burns. One school recommends early, repeated dilatation from above or retrograde if feeding gastrostomy has been done. Another school recommends conservative management by steroids and antibiotics. Steroids mainly inhibit scar formation later on due to their anti-inflammatory action. Antibiotics prevent infection.

- Diet has to be changed from liquid to semisolids gradually as the patient tolerates. If stricture forms despite repeated esophageal dilatation, a temporary feeding gastrostomy is done followed by definitive surgical repair of the stricture.
- Inhalational injury by exposure to chemical gases (e.g. ammonia) can cause respiratory distress. Fiberoptic bronchoscopy is helpful in establishing diagnosis. Management is the same as for inhalational injury otherwise (Fig. 10.5).

Chemical burns of eye (Figs 10.6A and B) can be very fatal so their diagnosis and treatment should be very prompt. Signs and symptoms of eye involvement are:

- excessive tears
- conjunctivitis
- blepharospasm

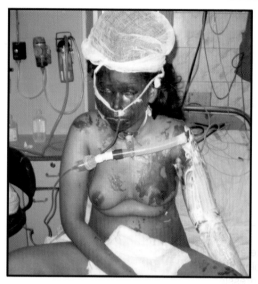

Fig. 10.5: Homicidal acid burns to face with inhalation and ingestion of acid requiring tracheostomy

- irritation in the eyes
- pupils may get semidilated and fixed.

Investigation: Slit-lamp examination or even a fluorescein staining can show signs of corneal involvement.

Treatment: is copious irrigation with water or normal saline till all the chemical has been diluted and removed.

Topical antibiotic drops to be used in case of proven corneal injury.

Prophylactic cycloplegics are used in case of danger of iritis.

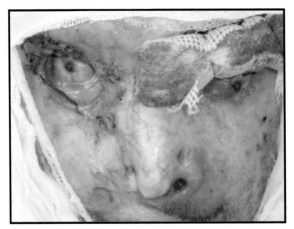

Fig. 10.6A: Acid burns to face involving both eyes. Right eye completely lost with total loss of upper lid with phthisis bulbi. Ectropion of left upper eyelid released and grafted with tie over stent dressing

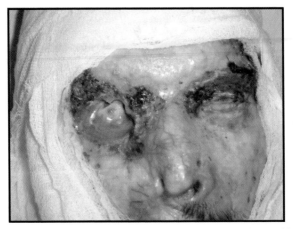

Fig. 10.6B: 1 week postoperative of same patient with grafted upper lid showing complete closure of left eye

Late complications of eye burns: Corneal ulceration, cataract, glaucoma, iridocyclitis and symblephron. Alkalis are more damaging to the eyes than acids because acids produce immediate precipitation of proteins which prevents further damage to the cornea, whereas in alkalis the hydroxide ion penetrates the cornea deep into the anterior chamber, eventually leading to pthisis bulbi.

SPECIFIC CHEMICAL BURNS

Sulphuric Acid

Uses: In laboratory, tanning industry and domestic use for toilet cleaning.

Mechanism of action: It is a dessicant and causes coagulative necrosis of skin and subcutaneous tissue.

Clinical signs: Depending on concentration and duration of contact it can cause deep dermal burns which present a bronzed leathery appearance or full thickness burns which produce a thick black eschar. Large burns can produce systemic acidosis.

Treatment: Copious irrigation with water till litmus test is negative, usually within 2 hours. In case of full thickness burns early excision and grafting is the treatment of choice (Figs 10.7A and B). In some places, a buffer phosphate solution containing disodium hydrogen and potassium di-hydrogen phosphate is used.

Hydrochloric Acid

Uses: In the laboratory.

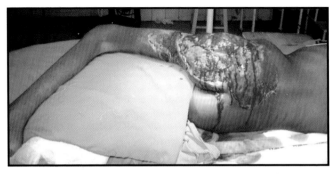

Fig. 10.7A: Raw area over buttocks and thighs following
deep burns by accidental alkali injury

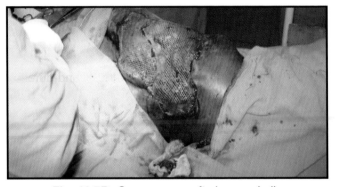

Fig. 10.7B: Same area grafted secondarily

Mechanism of action: It is a dessicant and also causes
coagulative necrosis of tissues. Reaction is slower but
deeper. In concentrated forms it can produce fumes which
if inhaled, can cause respiratory burns also.

Clinical signs : Yellow, brown discoloration of skin.

Treatment : As for all acids.

Nitric Acid

Uses: In laboratory and in jewellery industry for polishing.

Mechanism of action: It causes coagulative necrosis with protein precipitation. Fumes can also cause inhalational injury.

Clinical signs: There is orange,yellow discoloration of skin due to xanthoprotein reaction.

Treatment: Same as for all acids.

Hydrofluric Acid

Uses: As a metal and glass cleaning agent and for etching glass and silicon chips also in manufacture of Teflon and high octane fuel.

Mechanism of action: It is a strong inorganic acid. It's action is both due to hydrogen ions and fluoride ions. Hydrogen ion produces coagulative necrosis as in other acids. Fluoride ion is highly permeable through the cell membrane and acts a metabolic inhibitor. It also binds to calcium and magnesium in the cells leading to cell damage and releases intracellular potassium which irritates nerve endings leading to severe pain. Fluoride ion penetrates deeply resulting in liquifactive necrosis and deep ulcers.

Clinical signs: In case of dilute acid, deep dermal burns are seen as typical slate grey colour lesion. In case of full thickness burns by concentrated acids, there is a deep ulcer with thick white eschar.

The amount of pain the patient complains of is usually out of proportion to the area of burn.

It may even cause gangrene of fingers because of vasospastic action of fluoride ions.

Treatment: Acid should be washed off with water as quickly as possible, and then calcium gluconate gel (2.5%) is to be rubbed gently over the area for 15 minutes or till the pain subsides in order to convert the fluoride ion into an insoluble complex of calcium fluoride.

- If burn is caused by concentrated hydrofluoric acid then 10 percent solution of calcium gluconate can be injected under the eschar except in case of fingers where skin is tight and any injection may cause necrosis because of edema of tissue. In these cases, incision of affected area or removal of nail in case nailbed is involved and then irrigating the area with calcium gluconate.
- Other substances used for this purpose are 50 percent magnesium oxide, calcium chloride, magnesium sulphate paste or injection, sodabicarb solution and quaternary ammonium compounds. In case of larger burns, there may be hypocalcemia and hypomagnesemia for which slow IV calcium gluconate is given.
- If hydrofluoric acid is ingested, mouth should be washed liberally with water and then patient is made to drink milk.

Chromic Acid

Uses: In electroplating, dye industry and production of alloys.

Mechanism of action: Action is by the chromium ion Cr^{6+} which penetrates cell membrane and acts as oxidizing agent, changes to Cr^{3+} which binds to protein leading to coagulative necrosis. Since it causes no pain because of its anesthetic action, the burns may become full thickness.

Clinical signs: The burned areas have yellowish discoloration. Chromic ulcers (Chromholes) are deep ulcers which are painless with pus in center surrounded by peeled areas. The oral lethal dose is 6 gm.

Systemic effects: In the form of –acute gastritis, hemorrhagic nephritis with acute tubular necrosis, hepatic failure, central nervous system involvement, inhalational injury leading to bronchospasm, anemia and coagulopathy.

Treatment: Immediate copious water irrigation followed by phosphate buffer or 5 percent thiosulphate soaks helps in diluting the acid and converting hexavalent Cr^{6+} to Cr^{3+} which is less toxic.

Absorption can also be prevented by other topical chelating agents like calcium EDTA, ascorbic acid. The best way to reduce mortality in case of deep burns is excision of full thickness area and skin grafting. In case of impending renal failure, timely peritoneal and hemodialysis can be effective especially if done before 48 hours, because after 48 hours the chromic ion binds to tissue proteins.

Phenol (Carbolic Acid)

Uses: In laboratories, to carbolize wards and operation theaters as antiseptic agent, in sanitizers, disinfectants and deodorants and chemical peeling of face by plastic surgeons.

Mechanism of action : It is a weak acid which is a misnomer because it behaves like an alkali. It has corrosive action produced due to exothermic reaction, dehydration of cells and precipitation of proteins. It also gets absorbed into the circulation to produce systemic toxicity. If diluted with water, its absorption increases.

Clinical signs : It has a soapy feel and characteristic odor. Very often perineal burns are seen in hospital staff where phenol placed in bottles is accidentally used in the toilets. Superficial burns caused by phenol are whitish grey in color and deep burns are black. Most of them are painless because it destroys the nerve endings by demylinating the nerves, thus increasing the risk of deep burns.

Systemic effects: Depression of central nervous system, hypothermia, hypotension, hemolysis, arrhythmias, cardiac arrest, renal failure and jaundice.

Treatment: Copious lavage with water, preferably with a shower because small amounts of water can increase its absorption. The best solvent used for swabbing is 50 percent polyethylene glycol (PEG) solution. Others include propylene glycol, glycerol and soap or household vegetable oil. In case of deep burns, patient is taken to the operation theater immediately to excise and cover the area.

Formic Acid

Uses: In tanning industry.

Mechanism of action: It causes coagulative necrosis and inhalational injury by fumes.

Clinical signs: Deep ulcers and respiratory changes.

Systemic effects: Hemoglobinuria, kidney failure, liver failure and acidosis.

Treatment: In case of full thickness burns excision and grafting is required. Otherwise washing with copious amount of water and conservative treatment is sufficient.Respiratory care is given in case of inhalation injury by fumes.

Petrol

Mechanism of action: It is a hydrocarbon,used as a fuel. Burns occur during road traffic accidents either because of spillage of petrol over clothes which remain in contact with body for a long time or inhalation of petrol fumes. Usually causes superficial burns and rarely deep burns.

Clinical signs: Blistering and pink staining of skin is seen.

Systemic effects: Central nervous system depression, liver failure, renal failure, bone marrow suppression.

Treatment: Removal of clothing soaked in petrol and immediate washing with soap and water. Wounds are treated by exposure method. In case the agent is leaded petrol it contains tetraethyl lead which can get absorbed through the skin and cause lead poisoning. Tetraethyl is converted to triethyl lead which is absorbed by the red blood cells. Therefore the amount of absorption can be estimated by measuring the blood levels of lead. It gets excreted in the urine. Its management includes daily measurement of blood and urine levels of lead. Penicillamine is used as a chelating agent till the values return to normal.

Kerosene Oil

Causes a typical epidermal necrolysis in which there is bleb formation and extensive separation of superficial skin layers.

Lime

Uses: In industries.

In case of exposure to lime, forceps are first used to remove lime particles from the surface and then area is to be washed with large volume of water so that the effect of heat produced by exothermic reaction of lime with water is nullified.

Cement

Cement contains 64 percent of calcium oxide (quick lime) by weight. When this reacts with water it forms calcium hydroxide which is a weak alkali which usually causes contact dermatitis. But if contact is for a longer period (2 to 6 hours) it can lead to full thickness burns. It typically involves burns around ankles if there is spillage of wet cement over boots or over the knees in case of kneeling in wet cement for a couple of hours. Treatment is early excision and grafting for full thickness burns.

Caustic Soda (NaOH)

Uses: In industries for manufacturing washing powder, detergents and cleaning agents and paint removers.

Mechanism of action: Is by hydroxyl ions which saponify fats by liquefactive necrosis thus burrowing deeply in to the tissues. The process continues for a long period of time usually for hours so that the depth of injury is more. Corneal injuries are very severe because there is very little resistance to penetration by the hydroxyl ion.

Treatment: Immediate copious water irrigation. Usual end point of irrigation is decreased pain and negative litmus test. Alternately, phosphate buffer soaks can be used for atleast 24 hours with half hourly change.

Potassium Hydroxide

Used in alkaline batteries and burns occur due to leakage of batteries and body parts coming in contact with it. Similar effects as caustic soda.

Sodium

Uses: In manufacture of photoelectric cells and tetraethyl lead, as polymerization catalyst and as a coolant in nuclear reactors.

Mechanism of action: Is a very reactive substance. In contact with water it forms $Na + H_2O = NaOH + H^+$. The hydrogen gas ignites in air and therefore it produces both thermal and chemical burn.

Treatment: Not to pour water immediately. Instead first pick out the particles of sodium from the skin and then remove the remainder by jet stream of water so that even if the particles of sodium do ignite, the heat gets dissipated by the high pressure flow of water.

Potassium

Potassium burns are less common than sodium burns.

Uses: As a catalyst in condensation, polymerization and reduction procedures.

Mechanism of action: On skin is the same as that of sodium. It also forms a superoxide when it comes in contact with moist air by a exothermic reaction producing oxygen and hydrogen peroxide.

Treatment: Same as sodium.

Phosphorus

Uses : In fireworks factory, ammunition factory, insecticides and fertilizers.

Mechanism of action: It causes direct thermal and chemical burns to skin. It rapidly oxidizes to produce P_2O_5 by exothermic reaction and P_2O_5 then formed is hygroscopic and combines with water to form H_3PO_4 (phosphoric acid) which is very corrosive to the skin.

Systemic effects: Phosphorus and its derivatives are fat soluble so they are rapidly absorbed into circulation leading to hypocalcemia, CNS depression, hyperphosphatemia, ECG changes –ST elevation, prolonged QT interval and bradycardia, hepatic failure and acute tubular necrosis.

Treatment: If phosphorus is exposed to dry air it continues to burn so the effected area has to be covered with moist dressings or washed with water along with physically removing all phosphorus particles with the help of a metal forceps. Small particles may be detected by their typical phosphorescence seen if patient is taken to a dark room. 1 percent copper sulphate has been suggested to convert phosphorus to cupric phosphide which is seen as black particles which can be easily removed. However, copper sulphate is to be used in very small amounts because of its own toxicity and washed off immediately after use. If the particles are lodged deep into the skin the area has to be excised keeping it moist at all times, removed pieces of phosphorus are to be discarded carefully because of risk of explosion on exposure to air.

Ammonia

Uses: In agriculture industry as a fertilizer, for manufacture of nitrates, as a refrigerant, in manufacture of vitamins, drugs, synthetic textiles and quaternary ammonium compounds.

Mechanism of action: It is a colourless pungent gas. Stored at high pressure in liquid form. Forms an alkaline solution in contact with water. Cutaneous burns produced by it are usually superficial with erythema and blisters. It is extremely irritating to the eyes. Inhalational injuries due to ammonia gas are most severe as it causes severe laryngeal and tracheobronchial edema leading to respiratory obstruction or chemical pneumonitis.

Treatment: For cutaneous and eye burns –copious water irrigation is done. In case of inhalational injury mechanical ventilation or tracheostomy with bronchial lavage will be required.

Molten Metals

Molten metal burns are the commonest industrial burns. Usually involves iron, steel, brass or aluminium. Since iron and steel have higher melting points (1530°),burns caused by them are usually full thickness burns whereas Aluminium has a lower melting point (650°), it causes only deep dermal burns.

These burns are usually seen in moulders, casters, furnacemen and foundry workers wherein the feet are the most commonly involved. Usually the explosion is caused by even small amounts of water getting into the molten metal, thus spattering the molten metal over different parts of the body.

Clinical signs: Molten metal burns typically involve the dorsum of foot as full thickness burns.

Treatment: Ideal treatment for the full thickness burns is primary full thickness excision and grafting. Another method is conservative treatment. Since the burns are usually deep they would take months to heal. In case of aluminium molten metal burns which are deep dermal, tangential excision and skin grafting is preferred. If sole of foot is involved, it is to be treated conservatively as the sole skin is very thick and usually heals spontaneously. If full thickness of sole skin is involved, then it can be excised and grafted.

Hot Molten Materials

Usually include tar (Figs 10.8A and B), Bitumen or plastics. Their characteristic feature being that since these materials

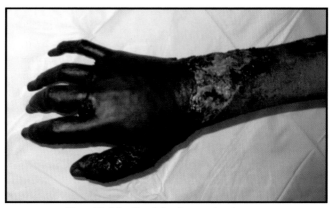

Fig. 10.8A: Coal tar burns to dorsum
of hand causing deep burns

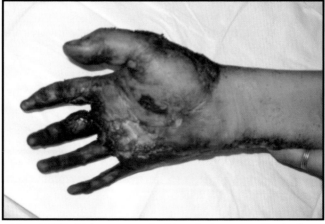

Fig. 10.8B: Palmar aspect of hand of same patient after
partial removal of coal tar with paraffin

adhere to the skin, the heat of the material continues to cause damage to underlying skin for a long time, thereby causing deeper burns than normally expected.

Treatment: Tar and Bitumen can be removed by applying any solvent material—most commonly used is liquid paraffin or even butter which are easily available. If removed in time, usually the burned areas heal spontaneously by conservative management.

In case of molten plastic burns, the plastic has to be removed surgically.

CHAPTER 11

Burns of
Special Site

Hands and face are the two practically always exposed areas of the body and these two parts of the body perform two very important functions. One provides the identity to the individual while other provides the livelihood, one is responsible for beauty while other is responsible for earning the bread. Destruction of one leads to unpresentable face, while destruction of other leads to loss of dignity- dependency on others and inability to earn one's livelihood or in other words converting the individual to a begging bowl!

Nearly in 80 percent of all extensive burns (burns more than 50%) either hand or face or both are involved. Nearly 70 percent of all OPD attendance of burns or smaller burns consist of either hand or facial burns. 90 percent of all burns admitted during Diwali days or cracker burns have burns of hand.

HAND BURNS

From functional point of view at the macro level hand burns are divided into two major groups:

1. Burns of hand only, i.e. hand burn is the major burn element.
2. Burns of hand along with other major burns of the body, i.e. hand burns is the minor burn element in total scenario of extensive life-threatening burns.

Saving life is always a priority over saving a hand. Hence where hand burns are in addition to the major burns of the body, aim is to avoid any further damage to the hand till definitive treatment is available for hand burns or in other words till other areas have healed/grafted.

In nearly 50 percent of the cases, resulting hand contracture is associated with other contracture of upper extremity like wrist, elbow and shoulder. Nearly 30 percent hand contractures have volar contracture. 20 percent have both volar and dorsal problem. 30 percent have dorsal contracture. 20 percent have major problems like loss of digits or phalanges.

Why hand becomes so deformed vis-a-vis other parts of the body? This is because of peculiar anatomic configuration and complex physiological function of the hand.

Anatomically hand consists of a single unit with whole of the upper limb. Hand which starts from the wrist forms a joint with lower end of radius and upper row of carpal bones and a joint with lower row of carpal bones and five metacarpal bones. In this only one joint the thumb carpometacarpal joint is important, as far as hand is concerned, as this is the joint which is responsible for opposition of thumb.

Metacarpals form important joints with the phalanges. These are the most important joints. MP joints of the fingers resemble to some extent to CMC joint of thumb as far as function is concerned. Relative importance of these two entirely different joints is same. IP joints though important have somehow least importance in relation to total hand function.

This basic building block is moved by complex system of extrinsic and intrinsic muscles. On the volar aspect this system is well protected by muscles, pad of fat and a thick layer of skin along with palmar fascia. Pad of fat is peculiar, i.e, each fat globule is surrounded by fibrous structure securing the fat globules between palmar fascia and deep layer of dermis. This system prevents any shearing movement between fat and skin. Whole system is like a Roho-cushion. On the dorsal side this system is less protective and that is the reason that maximum damage to these structures is seen in cases of burns.

Burns leads to edema and swelling of hand and to collect this maximum amount of fluid hand adopts the position of ease which consists of palmar flexion at wrist level, straightening of MCP joints and bringing closer 1st CMC joint (Figs 11.1A to C). Adoption of this position makes the hand non-working. This effect is further compounded by damage to the unprotected extensor apparatus, rupture of central slip and volar displacement of central slip. This leads to flexion at PIP joint which is compensated by hyperextension of the MCP joint and transmission of forces to DIP joints leading to hyperextension at DIP joints. This whole system of deformity is termed as the Boutonniere deformity. Sometimes direct damage to extensor tendon of DIP joint leads to mallet finger deformity. The adducted thumb adopts hyperextension at MCP joint and flexion at IP joint leading to Z deformity of thumb. The fusion of adjoining raw areas of the fingers leads to webbing, forming syndactyly or a mitten hand in worst cases. In the worst cases the fingers may be completely lost either by direct effect of fire or secondary effect of compression by swelling. This is the basis of complex post-burn deformity. Aim of the burn surgeon is to prevent, anticipate and quickly treat the problem and prevent any further damage (Figs 11.2A to 11.3).

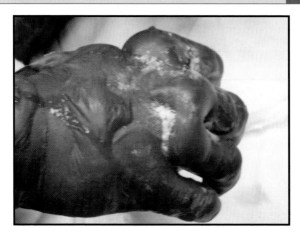

Fig. 11.1A: Superficial dermal burns to hand showing typical blisters

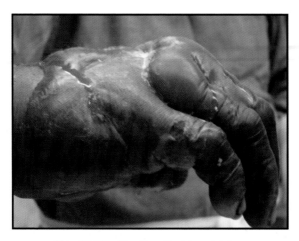

Fig. 11.1B: Position that hand takes after burns due to edema

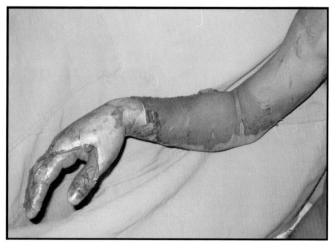

Fig. 11.1C: Same patient after removal of blisters showing typical features of superficial dermal burns –moist pink surface which blanches with pressure. Note the position of rest of the hand - flexion at wrist, which should be avoided during dressings

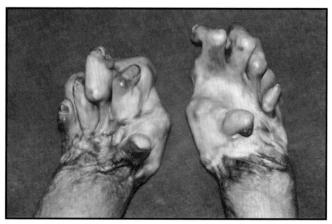

Fig. 11.2A: Severe post-burn contracture of both hands showing typical clawing of all fingers

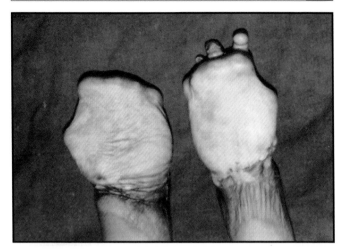

Fig. 11.2B: Same hands showing reversal
of metacarpal arch

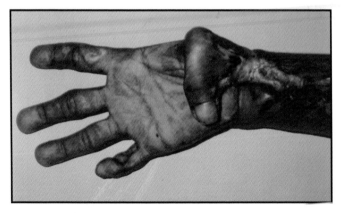

Fig. 11.3: Adduction contracture of thumb

In burns of hand alone definitive treatment is provided immediately and aim is to achieve full function of hand vis-à-vis in second group definitive treatment is delayed till patient is fully stabilized and risk to life has been fully averted. Aim for these cases is to avoid secondary damage, providing correct position so that even when no attention or least attention is given to the hand further damage is averted. Unfortunately this point is often neglected and is responsible for post-burn disabilities of the hand, thus these deformities are of secondary nature and occur during the most important period when one is struggling to save patient's life (Figs 11.4A to 11.7B).

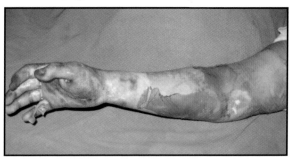

Fig. 11.4A: Circumferential deep dermal burn of hand and arm

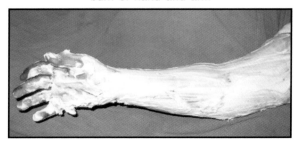

Fig. 11.4B: Silver sulphadiazine being applied to the wounds

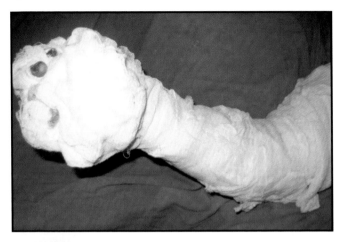

Fig. 11.4C: Gauze dressing done to cover the wounds with 'Ball' holding position of hand to maintain functional position

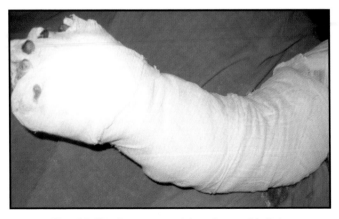

Fig. 11.4D: Gamgee and bandage with light compression tied over the dressing

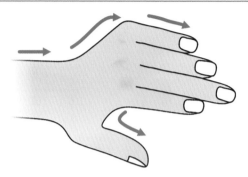

Fig. 11.5: Ideal hand position with extension at wrist, flexion at MCP joint and full extension at IP joints of all fingers and thumb in abduction with its MCP and IP joints in extension

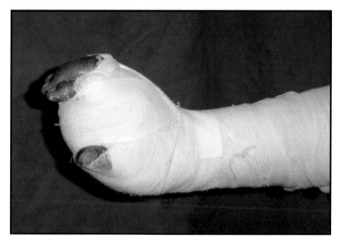

Fig. 11.6: Cock up position of hand in dressing maintaining the ideal functional position to avoid deformities

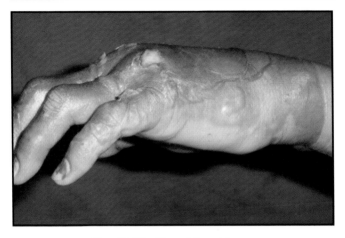

Fig. 11.7A: Dorsal hand burns

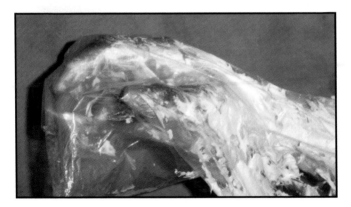

Fig. 11.7B: Same hand as in Figure 11.7A kept in a transparent plastic bag after applying topical antimicrobial cream to allow active movements of all joints

Table 11.1: Hand burn management

Hand burns alone
Volar

Superficial	Cock-up splint/full movements of the hands in gloves (Fig. 11.8).
Deep dermal	Cock-up splint/full movements of hands in gloves. Dynamic splintage for three months after healing Or Immediate shaving and grafting followed by dynamic splint for three months.
Full thickness	Immediate excision and grafting and splintage (static) followed by dynamic splintage for three months after healing.

Dorsal

Superficial	Cock-up splint/full movement of hand in gloves.
Deep dermal	Excision and grafting and splintage (static) followed by dynamic splintage for three months after healing.
Full thickness	Immediate excision and grafting (or flap) followed by dynamic splintage for three months.

Combined (Volar and Dorsal)

Superficial	Cock-up splint/full movements of hands in gloves.
Deep dermal	Excision and grafting and splintage (static) in straight position followed by dynamic splintage for three months after healing.
Full thickness	Excision and grafting and splintage (static) in straight position followed by

Contd...

Contd...

dynamic splintage for three months after
healing (Fig. 11.9).

Hand burns- along with other major burns
Volar aspect alone

Superficial

Hand rest with wrist in dorsi-flexion,
MCP 90° flexion, IP straight, thumb
abducted and extended-maintain the
position for 2 weeks — healed —
physiotherapy.

Deep dermal

Same as above-healed 3 weeks-
physiotherapy plus splintage.

Full thickness

Dress with the MCP's straight and fingers
abducted. Graft on granulating areas
after patient is stabilized — physiotherapy, Dynamic splintage for 6
months.

Dorsal aspect alone

Superficial

Dress as for volar aspect-healed- 2
weeks splintage.

Deep dermal

Fix MCP's in 90° with IP's straight with
K-wires—dress-healed 3 weeks—K-
wires removed-pressure garments with
intensive physiotherapy.

Full thickness

Same as above, grafting on granulating
areas/if patient stabilizes early and skin
is available-excision and grafting/ flap
cover-intensive physiotherapy.

Combined (volar and dorsal)

Same as above, only hand to be
maintained in neutral position during
waiting period.

If these principles are used judiciously bad deformities of the hand if not completely prevented, they are at least reduced to minimum.

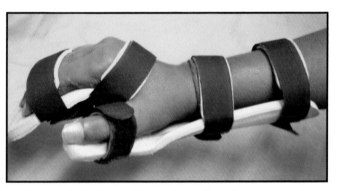

Fig. 11.8: Typical tailor made static splint to maintain position of all joints of the hand

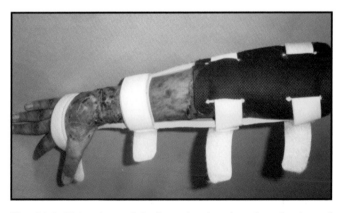

Fig. 11.9: Extension splint after releasing dorsal contracture of wrist and elbow to maintain extension and prevent dorsal contracture

FACE BURNS

Face is involved in one-fourth of all major burns. The outcome of face burns has significant aesthetic and social implications because a face which is the mirror of one's personality has been scarred for life, makes the patient most self conscious and hinders his social acceptability. Thus, though head and neck accounts for only 10 percent of TBSA in adults, in infants on the other hand it accounts for 19 percent of TBSA, face requires special attention.

Clinical problems associated with face burns (Figs 11.10 and 11.11).

- The possibility of inhalation injury should be always kept in mind in case of face burns as it effects the further management.
- Edema formation in face is always severe following superficial burns because the rich blood supply and loose skin of face allows for disproportionate fluid loss into this area.
- On the other hand in case of full thickness burns of face, the external edema may not be very apparent because of the thick eschar which inhibits fluid accumulation beneath it. Instead in these cases usually the fluid accumulates in the soft tissues of the oral cavity which can interfere with swallowing.

Why Face Burn is Given Special Consideration?

Mainly because healing in face is different from that of the rest of the body because of its rich vascularity. Also the number of epithelial appendages go deep into the

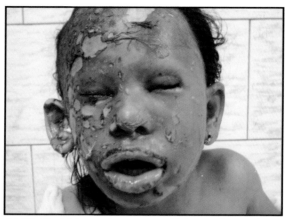

Fig. 11.10: Facial burns in a young girl due to fire cracker injury with mixed superficial and deep dermal burns. Note the intraoral edema

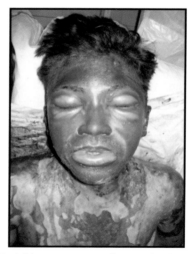

Fig. 11.11: Facial burns as part of extensive burns in a young adult with excess edema of face especially lids and lips

dermis in the facial skin so that the epithelialization is faster. This is true even if the burns are deep especially in males in whom because of the bearded skin, the epithelium lining the hair follicles which are embedded into dermis till different depths, regenerates fast enough to heal facial wounds.

The SMAS and platysma under the dermis of facial and neck skin also contracts in case of deep burns thus contributing to contractures following healing of deep facial burns. This presents in the form of ectropion of lips and lids and eyes.

Management for Face Burns

On admission of a patient with face burns the first step is to differentiate whether it is a case of face burns alone because of scalds or whether it is associated with inhalational injury also as is seen in most thermal burns.

The initial management for all facial burns includes washing of face thoroughly, clipping of facial hair in a bearded patient, debridement of loose dead skin, evacuation of blister fluid leaving its epithelium intact as a biological dressing.

The head end has to be elevated by 30° which not only makes a patient more comfortable facilitating respiration but also decreases edema formation by reducing the venous congestion of a dependent position.

In case of associated inhalational injury, if there are signs and symptoms of respiratory obstruction because of edema, which usually appears by 24 hours following burns, endotracheal intubation is done. In case intubation is difficult because of severe pharyngeal edema, tracheostomy should be the procedure of choice rather than causing trauma by forced endotracheal intubation which increases edema further, later on.If edema is not severe enough to demand intubation, patient is given humidified oxygen by mask and nebulization with saline or steroids.

Nostrils should be cleaned and lubricated with some ointment.

Eye care is given especially when there is edema of eyelids, by washing regularly with saline and instilling antibiotic drops and ointment.

Facial Burn Wound Management

At times it is difficult to differentiate between deep partial thickness and full thickness burns of face, especially in a bearded male. However, since facial healing is very fast and almost certain within 3 weeks, even in deep partial thickness burns, early excision and grafting is usually not done. A more conservative approach is followed for atleast 10 days. This can be done either by open method or closed method.

In closed method (Fig. 11.12) the entire face is dressed as in other part of body with paraffin gauze, antimicrobial cream, gauze and bandage leaving the eyes, nostrils and mouth open. However, these dressings are bulky and may interfere with movements of mouth. This causes restriction of oral intake by the patient and is more cumbersome and has no additional advantage over the exposed method.

Open method or exposed method (Figs 11.13 and 11.14) is therefore practiced in majority of the burn centers. This is in the form of applying a topical

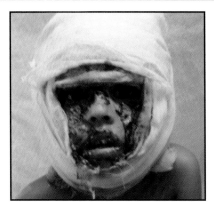

Fig. 11.12: Closed dressing method for face burns

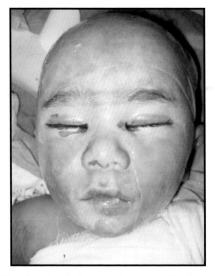

Fig. 11.13: Collagen sheet application in superficial dermal burns of face

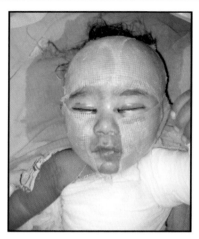

Fig. 11.14: Exposed treatment for face burns by applying paraffin gauze and antimicrobial ointment

antimicrobial ointment over the burned area rather than a cream base. This is left exposed to the air which has a drying effect on the wound thus inhibiting infection. Though a layer of crust may form over the area and healing by epithelization takes place under this layer of crust. The ointment has to be applied atleast twice a day so as to maintain lubrication over the wounds and over-come drying effects of air and inhibit bacterial colonization.

Some surgeons feel that the crust formation may serve as a culture media for bacteria and to inhibit formation of crust, moist dressings are applied to the facial wounds every 6 - 8 hours. In this one has to ensure that the dressing is kept moist always because moisture enhances epithelization though at the same time chances of bacterial colonization is increased. Biological dressing materials can also be used instead of routine dressings.

In case areas do not start healing in 10 days and it is established that they are deep burns which will require grafting, wet to dry dressing technique can be used over the necrotic tissue to remove the dead eschar and help in early appearance of granulation tissue. Once healthy granulation tissue appears, it should be immediately grafted.

If grafting is done, sheet grafts should be used without meshing (Figs 11.15A and B). It is preferable if sheets are applied as per the aesthetic units.

Ear Burns

In case there is involvement of ears also, patient is advised to use a donut to avoid pressure on the ears.The ears have to be managed by closed method (Figs 11.16A to D) by applying paraffin gauze, antimicrobial cream, filling up the grooves of the ear with cotton or gauze giving it a contour dressing.This is done to prevent edema of the skin of the ear which will separate the skin from the cartilage of the ear, thus hindering the blood supply of the cartilage (which comes from the overlying skin only). This promotes the development of chondritis and later on abscess formation, loss of cartilage and thus a deformed ear (Figs 11.17 to 11.19).

It is found that in facial burns involving the ears, 25 percent of the patients will develop chondritis of the ear.

Signs and Symptoms of Chondritis

Patient complains of throbbing sensation in these cases which is not relieved by analgesics.

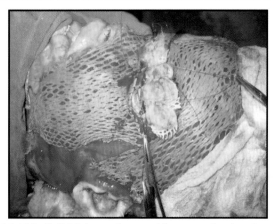

Fig. 11.15A: Full thickness burns of face –excised and meshed grafts applied to raw areas because of excessive bleeding which can lead to hematoma under the graft. Ideally meshed grafts are not preferred for face.The upper lid has also been released by excision of full thickness eschar and graft applied over it with a tie over dressing

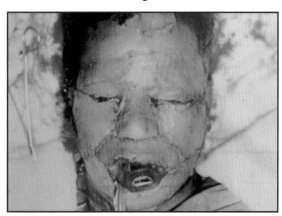

Fig. 11.15B: Unmeshed split skin grafts applied to the aesthetic units of the face in an another patient

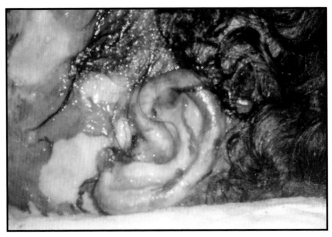

Fig. 11.16A: Superficial dermal burns
of ear along with face burns

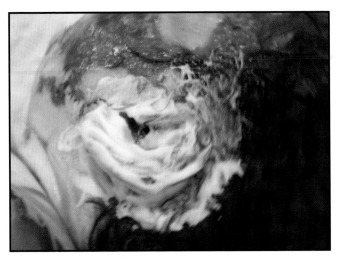

Fig. 11.16B: Ear covered with 1 percent SSD

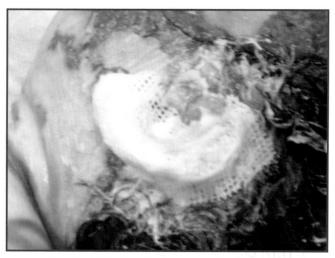

Fig. 11.16C: Paraffin gauze applied over ear

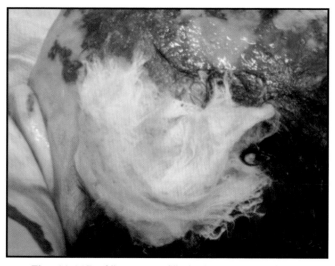

Fig. 11.16D: All grooves filled with cotton fluffs for
contoured dressing

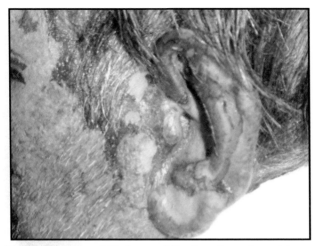

Fig. 11.17: Chondritis in ear following deep dermal burns with swelling, erythema and severe pain

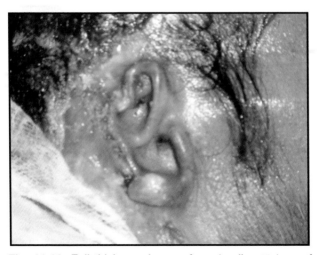

Fig. 11.18: Full thickness burns of ear leading to loss of cartilage and helix following acid burns

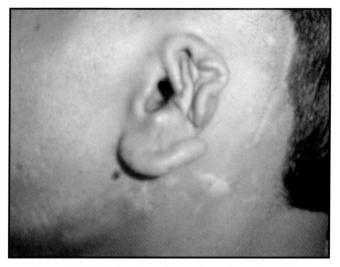

Fig. 11.19: Deformity of ears following chondritis

On examination the ear especially helix is swollen, erythematous and very tender. There is increase in the concho cephalic angle.

Treatment (Figs 11.20A to 11.21F): Early diagnosis is essential to relieve the patient of his pain. The only treatment is excision of involved cartilage which can be done bedside in case of critically ill patient or in the operation theater under local anesthesia. Incision is given along the helical margin to split the medial and lateral surface of ear and all the dead cartilage which is soft and yellow and inelastic is removed. The healthy cartilage which is pure white and elastic is left as such.

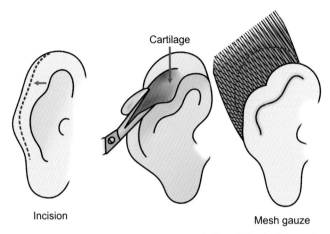

Fig. 11.20A: Stepwise management of chondritis. Incision given along helical rim. Dead cartilage exposed and excised. Space filled with mesh gauze

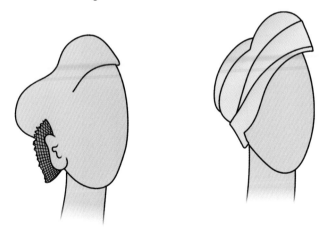

Fig. 11.20B: Light compressive contoured dressing over same ear

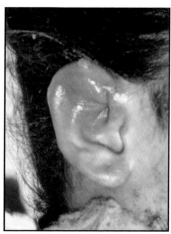

Fig. 11.21A: Typical picture of severe auricular chondritis with chondral abscess after burns of ear have almost healed. History of severe pain and on examination local swelling and erythema in upper half of ear with focal abscess about to burst open at one point

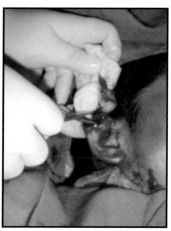

Fig. 11.21B: Incision given to drain abscess and remaining dead cartilage removed

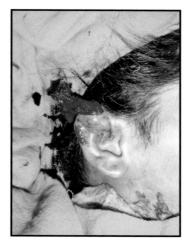

Fig. 11.21C: Dead space lightly packed with gauze

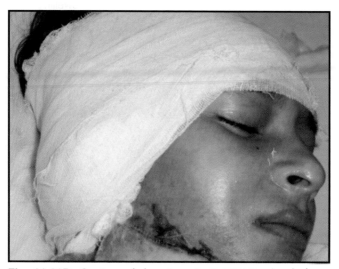

Fig. 11.21D: Contoured dressing given over the treated ear

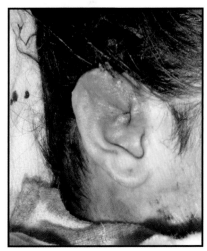

Fig. 11.21E: Forty-eight hours post-treatment picture with settled erythema and tenderness. Induration is much reduced

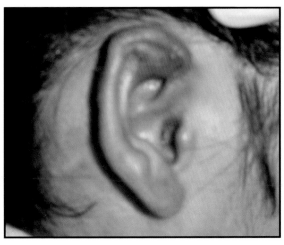

Fig. 11.21F: Two months post-treatment picture showing fairly well maintained contours

The cavity created is then packed with gauze and supporting the ear both on its medial and lateral surface with additional gauze, taking care not to fold the ear on either side. An occlusive dressing is given over this. The dressing is removed after 24 hours to re-examine the ear.

BURNS AROUND THE EYES (FIG. 11.22)

Direct injury to the eyes by flames are very rare because of reflex closure of lids which is a protective instinct. It is usually the skin of the lids which are involved. Though in case of acid burns and fire cracker injury the eyes are involved very commonly. Nevertheless, eyes have to be examined in all cases of face burns by the ophthalmologist.

Management

The first step in management is to irrigate the eyes thoroughly with saline or tap water especially if burn is by some unknown chemical. Burns caused by phosphorus require manual removal of particles. One should not wait for a specific antidote as acid base neutralization reaction is an exothermic reaction. And the heat liberated can worsen the damage already caused to the eyes by the chemical.

In thermal burns of face where the lids become severely edematous leading to closure of eyes, combination of antibiotic drops and ointment have to be instilled in both the eyes to prevent infection. Eye care is required every 4-6 hours by irrigating with saline to remove left over ointment and reinstalling drops or ointment. Once edema settles, ointment is discontinued.

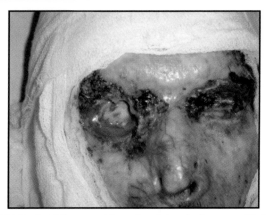

Fig. 11.22: Acid burns of face involving both eyes. Right eye shows complete loss of upper lid with phthisis bulbi. Left upper lid ectropion released to protect the eyeball and preserve whatever vision is left

Steroids are not indicated because they can promote bacterial infection and ulceration.

If there are deep burns of eyelids which causes retraction or eversion of lids to such an extent that the cornea remains exposed, special effort has to be made to protect the cornea. This is done by surgical release of the lid by excising the eschar and covering the raw area with a moderate thickness skin graft in upperlid and full thickness graft in lower lids.

Eversion of eyelids especially upper lid prevents normal moistening of cornea leading to drying of cornea which leads to corneal ulceration, perforation and ultimately blindness.

Another surgical option available for everted lids leading to corneal exposure is tarsorrhaphy. Though tarsorrhaphy is not practiced in all cases of lid retraction because of its potentially hazardous complication of damaging the edematous lid tissue. There are only specific situations in which tarsorrhaphy is indicated as in case where definitive grafting cannot be done as in extensive burns and cornea is very likely to get damaged.

Technique of Tarsorrhaphy (Figs 11.23A and B)

The opposing edges of the lids are denuded of epithelium at two places for a distance of 3 - 4 mm and these denuded areas are approximated by mattress sutures over a rubber bolster to prevent cut through of sutures. The suture usually used is Nylon 4 - 0. During this procedure one should ensure that the eyelashes do not get inverted and irritate the cornea. Later on, following this procedure, eyes have to be irrigated with saline every 12 hours and antibiotic drops instilled into the eyes.

In case of severe burns especially chemical burns in which the entire lid margin is destroyed and eyeball is exposed completely, conjunctival flaps can be used to cover the globes. In case whole of the lids are damaged, the conjunctival tissue is dissected from upper and lower lids and sutured together with an absorbable suture. This is covered with a skin graft.

In case of high voltage electrical injury, cataract formation is noticed hours to years after the injury.

In case there is a defect of corneal epithelium after acid or alkali burns, apart from saline irrigation for at least 30 min, other measures also have to be used. These include -cycloplegics - to decrease pain of iritis and topical antimicrobials - to decrease infection.

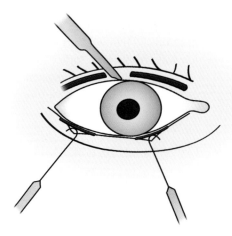

Fig. 11.23A: Line diagram showing steps of tarsorrhaphy. Upper and lower lid de-epithelialized at two places

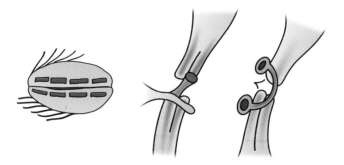

Fig. 11.23B: The two lids brought together to adhere the opposing raw areas with the help of bolster sutures

CHAPTER 12

Radiation Burns

Though radiation burn injury can manifest in different ways, civilian patients,who receive high doses of radiation for cancer treatment, are susceptible candidates for radiation burns or in soldiers accidental exposure occurs due to explosion of a nuclear device.

Mechanism of Action

1. *Thermal effect*: Is due to flash burns due to radiation heat from a detonation. These will produce superficial burns mainly.
2. *Radiation effects*: Is through intracellular damage by highly reactive chemical products including free radicals which are formed by transference of radiation energy (either through X-rays, gamma rays or neutrons or beta particles). Injury depends on — dose, wavelength and frequency of radiation. Long wavelength radiation is produced by radio waves, visible light and infrared light. It penetrates living tissue to a small depth and damage is due to heat produced by them. Radio waves do not cause severe injury except headache and weakness. Infrared waves may cause superficial burns and cataract.

   Short wavelength radiation results in very severe tissue damage due to ionizing effect. These include X-rays and gamma rays which penetrate deeply and can cause severe injury.

ACUTE RADIATION RESPONSE

Begins within hours of exposure in the following manner.

Prodromal symptoms: In the form of nausea, vomiting, diarrhea, fatigue, fever and headache.

Hematologic changes: Appear after exposure to 1 - 2.5 Gy. The tissue with maximum sensitivity to radiation is the bone marrow leading to pancytopenia. Granulocytopenia lowers the body's immunity making it more susceptible to infection.

Gastrointestinal changes: Appear with exposure to very high doses of radiation approximately 8 - 12 gy, presenting as nausea, vomiting, bowel cramps and watery diarrhea. The transport capability of the gut is reduced because of epithelial damage which promotes translocation of bacteria across the gut leading to sepsis.

Death is usually due to infection and hemorrhage.

Vascular system is also very susceptible to damage by high doses of radiation because of destruction of endothelial cells. Radiation usually effects the rapidly growing cells and since capillaries are most rapidly growing cells, the maximum damage by radiation is to the vascular system. Next most rapidly dividing cells are epithelial cells. Because of damage to capillaries and epithelial cells, wounds caused by radiation burns do not heal on their own and become chronic non-healing wounds. Since susceptibility of cells is proportional to their ability to divide, the least susceptible are the cells of the central nervous system.

Management

The victim has to be evacuated from the source and then assessed first for ABC (airway, breathing and circulation). The contaminated clothes have to be removed and area washed with soap and water. Next assessment for degree of thermal effect and radiation injury is done.

Thermal injuries have to be dealt with accordingly as in other thermal burns. Resuscitation steps are also the same. If there is diarrhea and vomiting, fluid loss need to be replaced accordingly. Signs of acute radiation syndrome have to be looked for. Hemoglobin, TLC, DLC and platelet count is done at regular intervals and blood and platelet transfusion is given depending on requirement.

Since immunosuppression is associated with radiation, the chances of infection are increased. Hence prophylactic antibiotics preferably in combination are to be started.

The administration of FFP, gammaglobulin, pentaglobin, etc. may help in improving the immune condition. If total body has been irradiated, bone marrow transplantation will be required between 3-5 days following exposure.

In case of radiation injury induced non-healing wounds, split skin grafting is not recommended as the bed is largely avascular. These conditions demand excision of wound with vascularized flap cover. This flap can be:

a. Free flap
b. Pedicled fasciocutaneous flap
c. Muscle flap.

CHAPTER 13

Physiotherapy in Burns

Physiotherapy is a very important tool in managing a case of burn from the first day itself.

Role of physiotherapy is:

- To control edema
- Maintaining range of movement
- Minimize scar formation using pressure techniques
- To make patient functionally independent
- To improve muscle strength and delay fatigue
- To resettle the patient in his occupation.

The physiotherapist has to gain trust and confidence of the patient and if the patient's family members provide support and participate in the patients physiotherapy program, it makes rehabilitation of the patient easier.

Physiotherapy in Acute Stage

Patient has to be seen by the physiotherapist from day one since by noting the areas of involvement the further treatment can be planned. The areas once dressed are usually not opened for the first 2 days. Apart from airway maintenance by well humidified air, the chest also needs special care as breathing control and relaxation techniques need to be established in order to avoid hyperventilation in a conscious patient. The head end of the patients bed is to be kept elevated so as to reduce edema in face and neck especially in face burns. Along with chest physiotherapy (Figs 13.1 and 13.2) the patient has to be taught to cough out expectoration on his own. For this, steam inhalation given twice a day is also helpful.

Since burned patient is in considerable pain, the first challenge faced by physiotherapist is to address the patients fear of moving a burned extremity because of anticipated

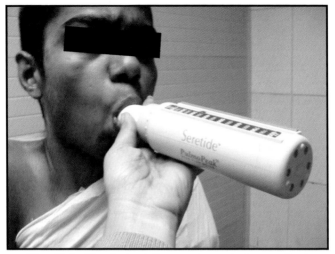

Fig. 13.1: Chest physiotherapy in acute burn patient

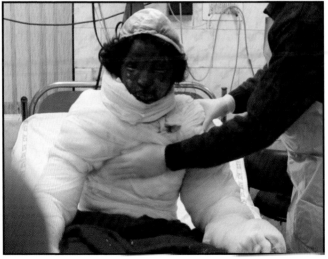

Fig. 13.2: Chest physiotherapy in acute burns

pain. In order to preserve the joint movements the edema has to be reduced quickly not only by proper resuscitation measures but also by elevating the extremities. Active movements have to be encouraged at the earliest. For this exposed method of treating the burn wounds of the extremities is a very good treatment option.

Exercises Indicated for Acute Stage

- Neck extension
- Trunk movements
- Knee bending and stretching
- Abduction of shoulder joint
- Elbow flexion and extension
- Pronation and supination of forearm
- Head rolling from side to side.

Thus active range of motion is encouraged at all joints. Repetitive exercises are done in opposite direction to that of the anticipated deformity. In the post-burn sequelae, contractures are the most common deformities which are of great concern to both the physiotherapist and the surgeon. Certain exercises and positions of joints can prevent formation of the contractures.

Joint	Position predisposing to contractures	Positions which prevent contractures
Elbow	Pronation and flexion	Full supination with extension
Shoulder	Adduction	Full flexion
Knee	Flexion	Full extension
Hand	Flexion of wrist and adduction of thumb	Extension and radial abduction of thumb
Foot	Plantar flexion	Dorsiflexion

Following healing of burn wounds, the deformities can be evaluated as follows:

- *Severe:* Where range of motion is only less than 50 percent of normal joint motion. For this reconstructive surgery is needed.
- *Functional:* Where 50 percent joint motions are preserved and patient can do his daily routine work.
- *Acceptable:* Where motion is limited in final arc of normal motion.

Orthoses: It is any device which when in contact with the body improves the function of that part.

Head and Neck

In the burns of anterior neck, neck is to be placed in extension by placing a small rolled towel behind the neck. Pillow is not recommended because it can cause contractures. A small "Donut" should be placed under the head in case of ear burns so that the ears do not rub against the bed.Cervical collar has to be applied to the neck over the dressing so as to avoid formation of neck contracture (Fig. 13.3).

Wrist and Hand Burns (Fig. 13.4)

In burns involving the dorsum of the hand, wrist is to be placed in dorsiflexion of 15° - 20°. with fingers flexed at MCP joint and IP joint in full extension with a support for the palmar arch. The thumb carpometacarpal (CMC) joint in between palmar and radial abduction with MCP and IP joint in extension. In case of burns involving only volar surface all joints are placed in extension and finger abduction.

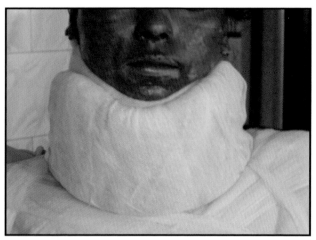

Fig. 13.3: Soft cervical collar to prevent anterior neck contracture. To be worn by the patient at all times

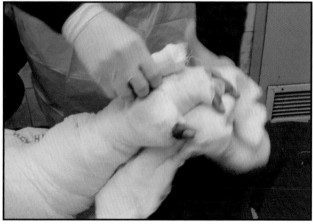

Fig. 13.4: Hand exercises done with dressing on and then splint tied again to maintain hand in position of function –wrist supported in dorsiflexion 15-20°, finger MCP joint in flexion, IP joint in full extension. Thumb carpo metacarpal joint in abduction and MCP and IP joint in extension

Elbow Burns (Fig. 13.5)

Elbow has to be placed in full extension with a well padded anterior or posterior splint.

Shoulder Joint

This joint has to be maintained in 90° abduction and external rotation by placing a wrist cuff which is then tied to a sling which then fixes to the head end of the bed. When the patient starts ambulating this can be given in the form of a tailor made airplane splint.

Hips

Are abducted to 15° to prevent maceration on inner thigh.

Lower Extremity Burns (Fig. 13.6)

In lower extremity splints are required for a longer period. The knee joint is in full extension and ankle in 90° flexion. During ambulation splints are to be worn during night only till patient is able to move his knees freely.

Ankle Burns

To prevent flexion contractures at the ankle, anterior ankle splints have to be worn by the patient. It helps in developing heel to toe gait. In case of burns on the posterior surface of ankles, they have to be kept in neutral position.

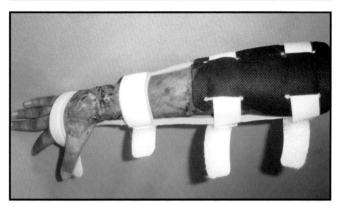

Fig. 13.5: Splint for volar surface burns of hand and forearm to keep all joints in extension and thumb in abduction

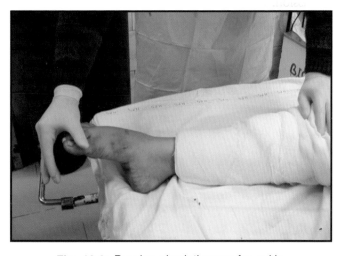

Fig. 13.6: Passive physiotherapy for ankle and legs in acute phase

Axilla Burns (Figs 13.7 and 13.8)

The axilla has to be maintained in abduction in order to avoid adduction contractures of the axilla. However if axilla burns are deep, grafting is required. The patient should be ambulated and made to use the other arm to support the operated one. Once the bandage is removed and graft is in place, exercises of the shoulder must be started. This is essential because the shoulder tends to become stiff in a cast or splint.

Splints

The positions of the joints can be maintained by splints. It is necessary to assess the need for splints just after admission. The type of splint will depend upon the extent and depth of burn. A splint will be required wherever the burned area crosses a joint.Splints are used both in acute stage as well as after grafting of raw areas or release and grafting of contractures (Figs 13.9 to 13.11).

Action of splint is to:
- Prevent contractures
- Prevent deformity
- Protect joints
- Protect newly grafted areas.

Types of Splints

Static splint - this maintains the effective body part in a fixed functional position.

Dynamic splint - a dynamic splint will substitute for weak or non functioning muscles or nerve injury

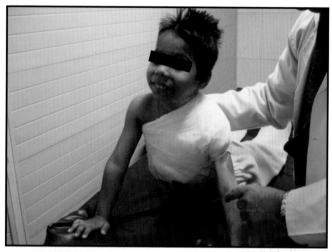

Fig. 13.7: Exercises for axilla and shoulder burns

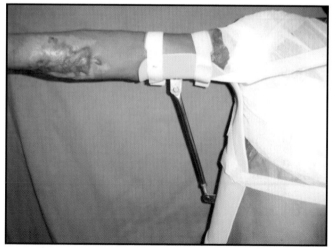

Fig. 13.8: Splint for axillary burns to maintain axilla in abduction and gradually increasing the angle of abduction

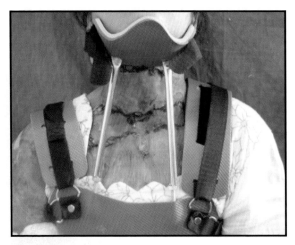

Fig. 13.9: Four post-cervical collar for released neck contracture to maximize neck extension

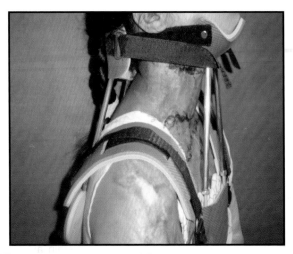

Fig. 13.10: Lateral view of four post-collar –rigid splint

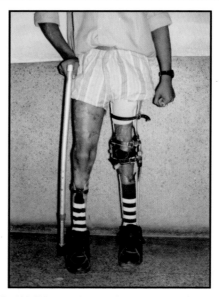

Fig. 13.11: Walking calipers for patient with paraparesis following spinal injury due to fall after contact with high voltage wire. Patient improved drastically with proper exercises

Each splint should be tailored according to need. Broad areas of contact will minimize and distribute pressure thus avoiding tissue necrosis. Positioning devices are employed as early as possible and used throughout the recovery period. Devices may be discontinued when full range of motion returns. Splint material should be non toxic and non-absorbent to avoid bacterial growth. Pre-fabricated light weighted aluminum splints are good in the beginning but they may not sustain the proper position for a long period. Plaster of Paris splints are cheap but absorb serous material and are not malleable once cured.

Hand Care

In case of hand burn, if proper care is not given the deformities can be very severe. The various hand deformities following burns of hand are as follows:

Claw Hand

Is characterized by extension of metacarpophalangeal (MCP) joints and flexion of interphalangeal (IP) joints and adduction of thumb. This results in loss of grip and pinch resulting in loss of nearly 60 percent of hand function. Contractures can be minimized if splinting is done from the beginning followed by exercises (Fig. 13.12). In the acute stage no passive movements are allowed so that rupture of all soft tissues is avoided.

A simple static splint provides flexion at MCP joint and extension at the IP joint. Thumb is maintained in abduction. Following grafting patient can be given pressure garment and splint to maintain the position of hand. Exercise is given to hands 2 - 3 times a day. Once the area heals completely, the patient must be encouraged to use the hands ensuring no further injury (Fig. 13.13).

Swan Neck Deformity

The contracture of intrinsic muscles cause flexion at MCP joint, hyperextension at proximal IP joint and flexion at distal IP joint. Early use of splint and exercises are needed.

Subluxation of MCP Joint

This may cause tearing or herniation of head of metacarpal or base of phalanx. Extension of MCP joint may affect

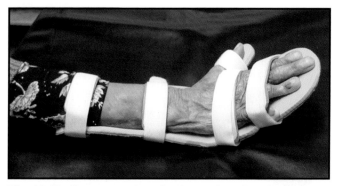

Fig. 13.12: Custom made splint for each patient according to specific deformity, is fabricated to counteract the forces of the deformity. Here the splint is preventing flexion at IP joint and hyperextension at MCP joint (Boutonneir's deformity)

the grip of the hand. The rehabilitation of this hand consists of splinting of MCP joint using a static splint initially followed by use of a functional splint for a few weeks accompanied by massage and exercises. Active exercises are recommended and the patient must be encouraged to start performing his normal tasks as early as possible.

Mallet Finger

Is caused by rupture or tear of extensor tendon proximal to the insertion of lateral band upon proximal aspect of the distal phalynx. Resultant damage allows the horizontal proximal pull of the extensor tendon and flexor digitorum profundus tendon causing loss of extension of distal phalanx.

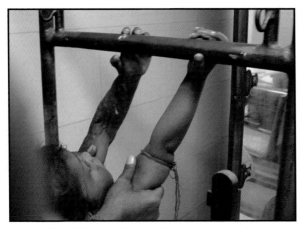

Fig. 13.13: Active assisted exercises for upper extremities following grafting

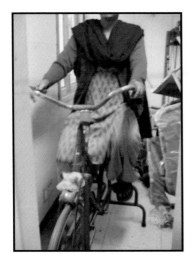

Fig. 13.14: Cycling for exercise of lower leg following healing of all wounds

Preventive Steps for Deep Vein Thrombosis

Burn patients especially in extensive burns are very susceptible to development of deep vein thrombosis because of:

- Increased viscosity of blood
- Increased coagulability of blood
- Immobilization due to pain.

Therefore special precautions have to be taken to prevent this complication. This can be done by early mobilization especially the lower limbs and ankle and knee exercises and elevation of legs in case they are also burned, in order to avoid stagnation of blood flow (Fig. 13.14).

CHAPTER 14

Post-burn Sequelae

The post-burn sequelae are usually in the form of scars and contractures. Majority of the burn wounds heal by scars except if it is a superficial or epidermal burn. These scars can be either well settled scars or can be hypertrophic scars or keloids. This depends on the:

1. *Depth of burns:* Deeper burns heal by hypertrophic scarring.
2. *Time taken for healing:* The longer the wound takes to heal, the more the hypertrophy.
3. *Surgical intervention:* It allows early wound closure and hence prevents the formation of hypertrophic scars and contractures.
4. *Color of skin:* By and large, the darker skin patients as in India and Africa, have a genetic tendency for hypertrophy of scars and keloid formation.

The burn scars have following characteristics (Figs 14.1 and 14.2):

1. *Vascularity:* Healed burn wounds are usually vascular and thus red in colour. If this redness settles in 2 months, there is usually no hypertrophy. But in case the scar shows evidence of increased vascularity even at 2 months, it tends to hypertrophy later.
2. *Hypopigmentation and hyperpigmentation:* Initially the scars are hypopigmented because of loss of melanocyte producing cells but the pigmentation is regained in few months. Later on most of the scars show hyperpigmentation especially in dark skin patients.
3. *Contractures due to fibroblasts and myofibroblasts and collagen:* There is an increase in number of fibroblast and myofibroblast in burn scars. As the myofibroblast in the wound bed contracts, it decreases the wound

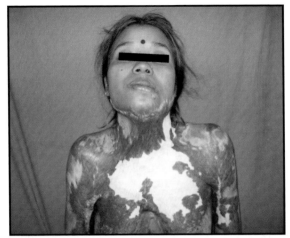

Fig. 14.1: Hypertrophic, hypopigmented and hyperpigmented scars following spontaneous healing of deep dermal burns with contracture of neck and both axilla

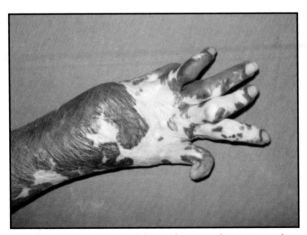

Fig. 14.2: Hypertrophic and hypopigmented scars on dorsum of hands causing deformity of all fingers and thumb

size to allow early closure of the wound by migrating epithelial cells which later manifests as contracture thus distorting the facial structures and joints.This pull by contracting myofibroblast may be sufficiently high to even dislocate joints as in case of MCP joints with scars of dorsum of hand, leading to reversal of metacarpal arch. The position of comfort for all joints is to be in flexion which if not prevented will permit new collagen fibers in wounds to fuse together and thus cause flexion contractures.

4. *Hypertrophy of scars*: It is the greater amount of collagen formation and alignment of collagen bundles that results in hypertrophy of scars. After some time, the scars mature with reabsorption of collagen.

Guidelines for Prevention of Hypertrophy and Contractures

There are certain prerequisites for prevention of hypertrophy of scars and formation of contractures. These are:

1. Proper positioning of body parts in the acute stage.
2. Use of splints to maintain proper position of all joints.
3. Exercises to keep joints supple.
4. Use of skeletal traction to maintain joint position if exposure method of grafting is used.
5. Following healing of wounds, use of pressure garments and splints.
6. Early maturation of scars by use of silastic gel sheets, massage and pressure garments.

Guidelines for Nonsurgical Treatment of Scars

Following healing of burn wounds till such time that the scars mature which may take 3 months to 3 years, special care of the scars should be taken in the form of massaging the scars, constant pressure and splinting.

Pressure garments (Fig. 14.3) have to be custom made and properly conforming whether it is for face or neck or extremities. Over the pressure garments splints made of orthoplast have to be applied. These have to be worn at all times during day and night except when massaging and exercising. Role of pressure garments can be explained by the following:

- They exert a pressure which exceeds the capillary pressure, i.e > 25 mm Hg. This helps in reducing the vascularity.
- They decrease the partial pressure of oxygen in the tissues.
- Decrease the amount of mucopolysaccharides.
- Decrease collagen deposition.
- Along with splints they oppose the forces of myofibroblasts and voluntary muscle action.

The scars need regular *massaging* (Fig. 14.4) with some oil to lubricate the skin as the skin in these areas tend to dry up because of absence of sebaceous glands in the scar tissue. In addition, steroid injection can be used intralesionally into the scars to soften them. Triamcinalone injection is used most commonly by dermajet syringe. This is repeated at 3 weeks for 4 months. Care is to be taken not to inject under the scar into normal tissue because that can cause fat atrophy. The advantages of steroid injections are:

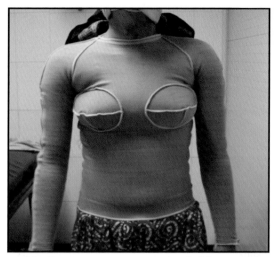

Fig. 14.3: Constant pressure on healed burn scars can markedly decrease hypertrophy and contractures

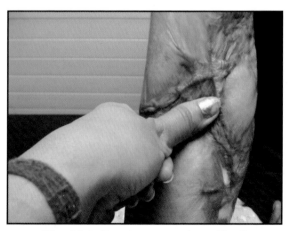

Fig. 14.4: Regular massaging with oil also allows scar maturation

- Early maturation of scars thus helping them to settle.
- Decreases pain in scars.
- Decreases itching in scars.

Silastic gel sheets also helps in early maturation of the scars. Giving ultrasonic diathermy is found to reduce the itching and tingling in scars (Figs 14.5 and 14.6).

Surgical Treatment of Scars and Contractures

Indications for Surgery

Surgery is indicated only once the scars have matured and are not in the active phase, which is indicated by decreased redness, absence of blanching in scar and decreased itching. Exceptions to this, when the surgeon is compelled to operate early, is when there is contracture causing severe functional problems as in contracture hands, ectropion of eyelids.

The various modes of treatment for post-burn hypertrophic scars and contractures are:

1. Serial excision of scars.
2. Z-plasty for contracture bands.
3. Full thickness excision of scars and skin grafting over healthy fascia.
4. Shaving of hypertrophic scars till healthy dermis and skin grafting over the reticular dermis which is unaffected by the burns (Same principle as in Tangential excision and grafting).
5. Release of contractures and skin grafting.
6. Release of contracture and flap cover.
7. Use of tissue expanders to advance the adjacent skin after excision of scar.
8. Bi-pedicle release of contracture and skin grafting on either side.

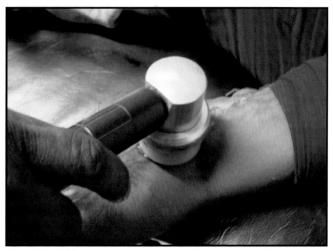

Fig. 14.5: Ultrasonic waves also used for hypertrophic immature scars which are believed to settle the scars faster

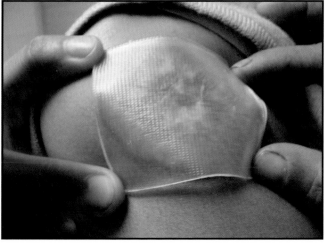

Fig. 14.6: Silastic gel sheet over immature scars

Scalp

Burns in the scalp usually cause alopecia without any scar hypertrophy or contractures because of immobility of skin and no tension from any side.

Surgical Options

- For small areas of alopecia either excision and primary suturing or serial excision at intervals of 3 months. Though the galea limits the elasticity of the scalp, multiple releasing incisions in the galea allows advancement of normal scalp over the excised area. This method can deal with alopecia of only one-third of surface area of scalp.
- If half or more than half of scalp is scarred, either rotation flap of hair bearing skin is moved anteriorly to give anterior hair line or tissue expanders (Figs 14.7A to 14.8D) are placed under the normal surrounding skin to expand it sufficiently to cover the alopecic patch completely.
- Hair transplant is not very useful in scarred skin, though if the scarred area has sufficient blood supply and sufficient thickness of subcutaneous tissue to support the transplanted hair follicles, hair transplantation can be tried.

Face

Surgical correction of facial scars and contractures is most difficult because of multiple areas of functional importance in the face, apart from the aesthetic aspect.

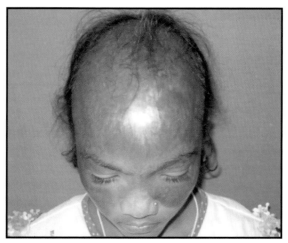

Fig. 14.7A: Post-burn alopecia over 2/3rd of scalp

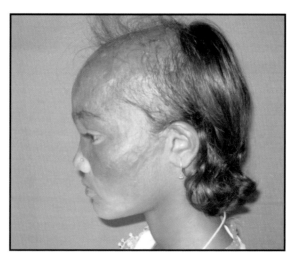

Fig. 14.7B: Lateral view of same patient showing only posterior half of scalp hair are normal

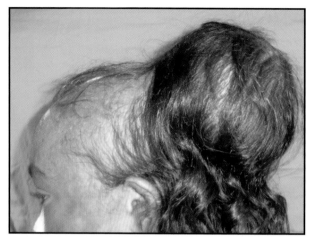

Fig. 14.7C: Tissue expansion of normal scalp

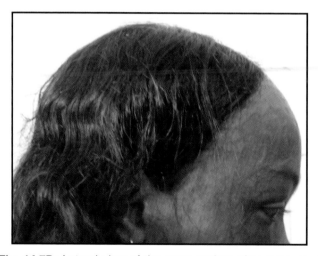

Fig. 14.7D: Lateral view of the same patient after removal of the expandor and anterior transposition of the expanded scalp

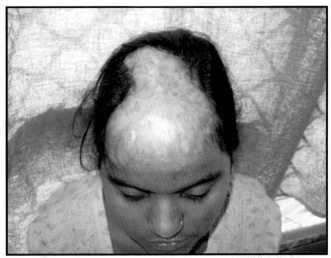

Fig. 14.8A: Post-burn alopecia of anterior and middle scalp

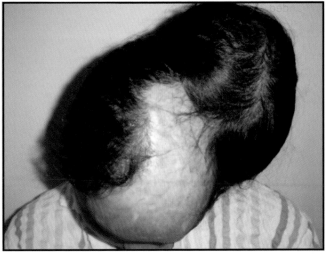

Fig. 14.8B: Tissue expander in normal scalp

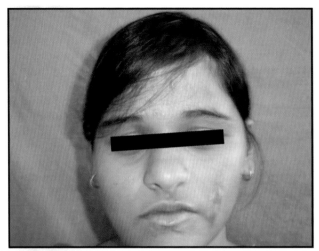

Fig. 14.8C: Anterior view of the same patient after removal of expander and of scarred scalp and anterior transposition of expanded scalp

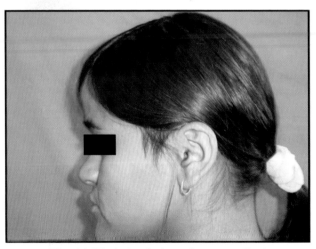

Fig. 14.8D: Lateral view of same patient

General Principles for Reconstruction of Face (Figs 14.10A to 14.11B)

- Avoid tension in certain areas since the facial features can get easily distorted.
- Grafts have to be placed within the limits of aesthetic units of the face (Fig. 14.9).
- Use moderate thicknes grafts from sites closer to the face so as to get a good color match, e.g. from post-auricular skin for full thickness grafts and upper arm for split skin grafts.
- Ectropion of eyelids has to be given top priority in order to protect the cornea and prevent keratoconjunctivitis.
- Flaps are not to be used for resurfacing the face because they become bulky and the facial expressions are lost.

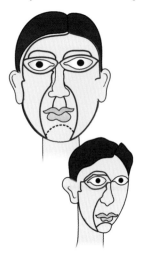

Fig. 14.9: Aesthetic units of face

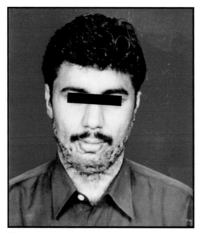

Fig. 14.10A: Severe post-burn hypertrophic scarring of bearded region of face and neck with embedded hair and micro-abscess formation

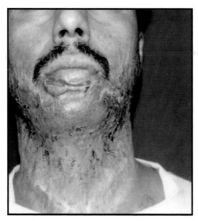

Fig. 14.10B: Postoperative picture of same patient following shaving of hypertrophic scar with Humby's knife till healthy reticular dermis over which split skin graft is applied

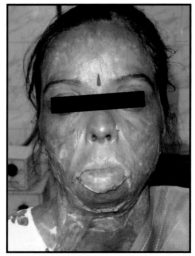

Fig. 14.11A: Severe lower lip ectropion and scarring

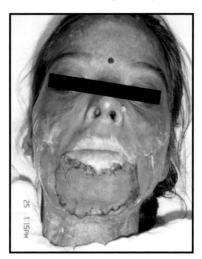

Fig. 14.11B: Excision of scar and grafting in aesthetic unit

Eyelids

The main aim of correcting deformities of eyelids is not only to restore appearance but also to preserve the functional integrity. The ectropion of lids can be:

a. Primary because of scarring of the lids itself or
b. Secondary because of the pull by scars of adjacent skin of face with normal skin of the eyelids.

Usually in case of ectropion of lids, the reflex Bell's phenomenon protects the cornea but if left for long, the other problems of conjunctivitis, pterygium, continuous tearing, etc. will continue and can be very irritating. Between the two lids, the upper lid ectropion needs to be released first and defect covered with moderate thickness graft because mobility of the lid has to be maintained. For lower lid ectropion, the defect has to be covered with full thickness graft because stability of lower lid is more important than movement (Figs 14.12 and 14.13).

Procedure: Releasing incision is given parallel and 3 mm away from the ciliary margin and contracture is released till the point of overcorrection for upper lid so as to compensate for postoperative graft contracture. Medially incision extends 5 mm beyond medial canthus and laterally 15 mm beyond lateral canthus. Grafts are sutured to the wound margins and fixed with a tie over dressing.

Eyebrow loss can be complete or partial. Surgical options are:

1. Free hair grafts from scalp (Figs 14.14A to C).
2. Pedicled graft based on branch of superficial temporal vessels. The graft is procured from the posterior scalp

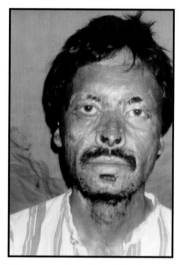

Fig. 14.12: Post-burn scarring face showing ectropion of upper and lower lid right eye and released grafted upper and lower lid left eye. Medium thickness skin graft used for upper lid and full thickness graft for lower lid

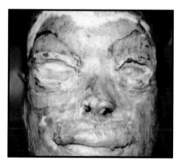

Fig. 14.13: Released and grafted bilateral upper lid, lower lid and upper lip. 1 week post of picture. Though there are bilateral corneal opacities, patient can now be taken up for corneal transplant

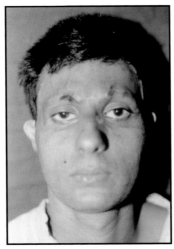

Fig. 14.14A: Post-burn loss of bilateral eyebrows

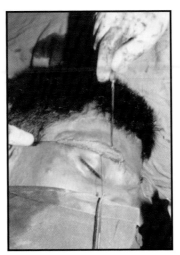

Fig. 14.14B: Eyebrow reconstruction with free composite hair graft from posterior scalp

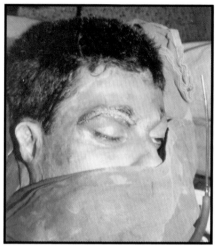

Fig. 14.14C: Postoperative picture of same patient with fully taken up hair graft

and shape has to match the shape of the eyebrows and direction of the hair should be upwards and laterally. The edges of the graft have to be beveled outwards to avoid cutting the hair follicles along the edges.

Ears

- Hypertrophic scarring of the helical rim requires excision and primary closure if cartilage is normal.
- If there is loss of cartilage and skin is crumpled up it has to be opened up and local flap is used to recreate the shape of the ear. Conchal cartilage graft from the other ear can be used to give the ear its proper shape.

- In case of partial loss of ear, upper one-third or middle or lower third, partial reconstruction with autogenous cartilage (from ribs or concha) with flap cover is useful.
- Complete loss of external ear is seen following acid burns of face. Though prosthetic ear can be one of the choices, the other alternative is total surgical reconstruction. Surgical reconstruction is a multistage procedure and is done using autogenous tissue (costal cartilage to carve a framework) which is covered with temporoparietal fascia over which split skin graft is applied. Surrounding skin is usually scarred or grafted so it cannot be used for reconstruction.

Nose

- Hypertrophic scars on dorsum of nose can be excised and resurfaced with split skin graft. If entire nose is destroyed, the forehead or arm tube flap is used to reconstruct the nose in stages, with costal cartilage for support (Figs 14.15A and B).
- In case the nostrils are stenosed due to burns, they can be opened up by 'Starplasty', in which two incisions perpendicular to each other are given in skin and mucosa to raise 4 skin flaps and 4 mucosal flaps. The skin and mucosal flaps are then interposed with each other in the form of a star to achieve a good nostril opening. Hence, this procedure has been given the name of starplasty (Figs 14.16A to 14.17B). The main advantage of this procedure is that it not only gives a wide opening but the interposed flaps break the scar line, thus preventing the scar contracture. Therefore the chances of restenosis are minimized. No postoperative splintage is required as no graft is applied.

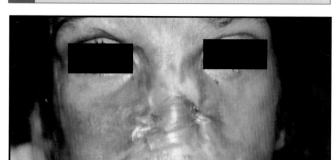

Fig. 14.15A: Total loss of nose with nostril stenosis and severe ectropion of lips

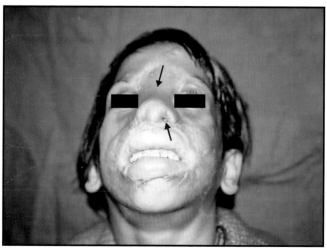

Fig. 14.15B: Nose reconstructed with arm tube and nostrils created by starplasty

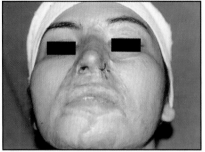

Fig. 14.16A: Post-burn scarring face with stenosed left nostril

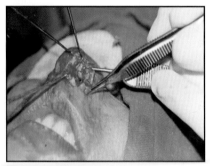

Fig. 14.16B: Preoperative picture with raised mucosal and skin flaps

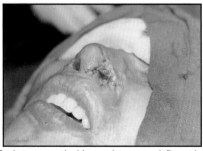

Fig. 14.16C: Interposed skin and mucosal flaps in the form of a star, hence given the name 'starplasty', creating adequate sized nostril opening. There is no need for postoperative splintage

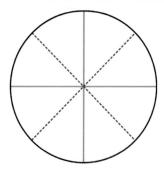

Fig. 14.17A: Line diagram for starplasty. Red lines indicate skin incision and green lines indicate mucosal incisions

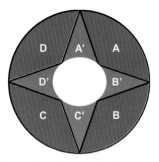

Fig. 14.17B: A, B, C, D indicate skin flaps interposed with A', B', C'and D' mucosal flaps creating an opening in the center. The shape resembles a star

Mouth

• Small scars around the mouth can be excised and primary closure with proper alignment of vermillion border can be done.

- In case of microstomia which can be severe especially following acid burns, the angles have to be released by Y to V plasty. It is important to release microstomia early under local anesthesia, because it restricts the oral intake and makes intubation difficult during anesthesia for other surgical procedures (Figs 14.18A and B).
- In case of ectropion of lower lip because of scar contracture of surrounding skin, there is too much of exposure of the normal red mucosa which causes drooling of saliva and food. This can be corrected by release of the ectropion at the vermillion border and resurfaced with thick skin graft. Best results are obtained if entire lower lip and mentum are resurfaced as an aesthetic unit after de-epithelializing the scar over the mentum. This avoids a flat look to the chin over the mentum (Figs 14.19A to C).
- In ectropion and scar of upper lip, releasing incision is given in the line of vermillion, maintaining a cupid's bow. The scar in upper lip is excised completely except in the philtrum which is only de-epithelialized. The skin graft placed in the philtrum is fixed with a tie over dressing to simulate the indentation.

Neck

- In mild neck contractures with simple contracture bands, correction is done by multiple Z - plasties or advancement flap from adjacent normal skin.
- In severe neck contractures, treatment of choice is release and thick split skin graft which is fixed with tie over dressing. The lateral extent of the incision is the

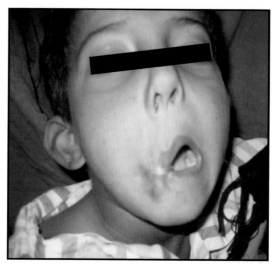

Fig. 14.18A: Scar contracture in the corner of the mouth following electric burns in a young boy causing microstomia

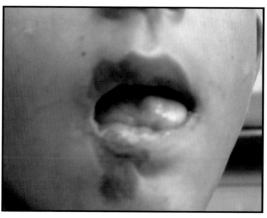

Fig. 14.18B: Release of contracture using cheek mucosal flap and tongue flap

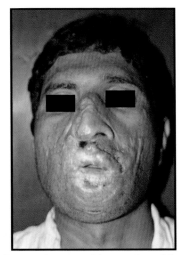

Fig. 14.19A: Severe hypertrophic scarring chin, upper lip and nose following acid burns with completely stenosed nostril and severe microstomia

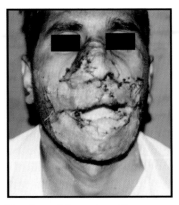

Fig. 14.19B: Shaving of hypertrophic scars and release of microstomia and skin grafting in first stage. In second stage, expander was placed in neck

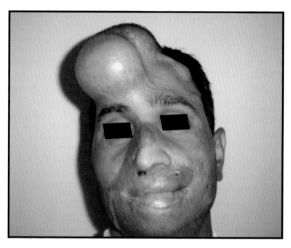

Fig. 14.19C: Third stage –Removal of expander from neck, excising scar from chin and transposing the expanded neck skin superiorly to bring normal bearded skin in chin and cheek. Reusing the same expander in the same sitting by placing it in forehead and scalp and using this expanded forehead for nose reconstruction

neutral line and the incisions are ended in a Y (fish tailing/dove tailing), to avoid linear contractures of the graft later on. Postoperatively the neck is kept in hyperextension by placing a pillow under the shoulders. After the graft settles, an orthoplastic splint is worn for 6-12 months to prevent recontracture. Flaps are not used for resurfacing released necks because they are bulky, they do not give a good cervicomental angle and give a poor aesthetic look (Figs 14.20A to 14.23D).

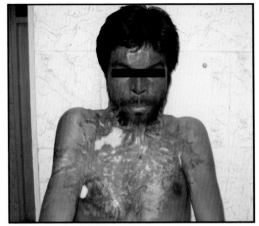

Fig. 14.20A: Hypertrophic scarring to chest and neck causing severe flexion contracture of neck and bilateral axillary adduction contracture

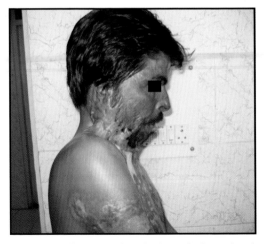

Fig. 14.20B: Same patient in lateral view showing loss of cervicomental angle

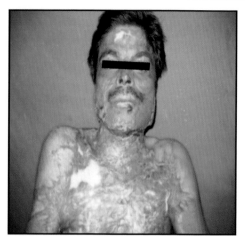

Fig. 14.20C: Postoperative picture of same patient with neck released and grafted to overcome functional deficit

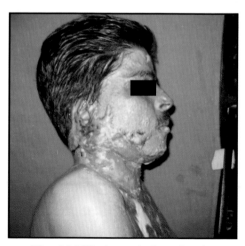

Fig. 14.20D: Lateral view showing restored cervicomental angle

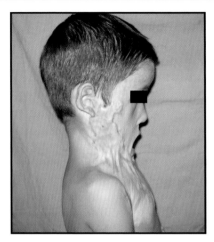

Fig. 14.21A: Four years old child with severe post-burn contracture (PBC) neck with ectropion lower lip with loss of cervicomental angle with severe functional restriction

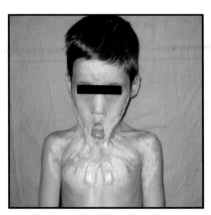

Fig. 14.21B: Anterior view of same patient.These patients require early reconstruction because the deformity interferes with speech, feeding and growth

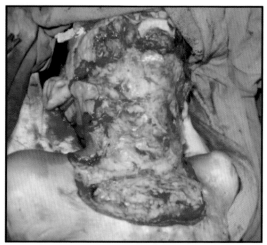

Fig. 14.21C: Excision of scars with complete release of contracture neck and ectropion lip

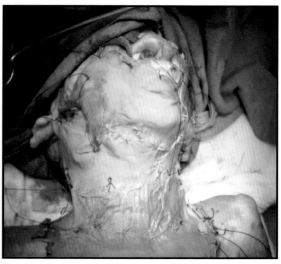

Fig. 14.21D: Skin graft applied to raw areas neck and chin

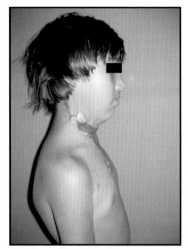

Fig. 14.22A: Mild contracture of neck in a young girl with obliteration of normal neck contour

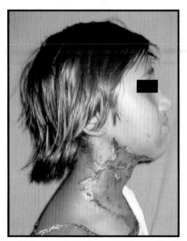

Fig. 14.22B: Released and grafted neck showing good neck and chin contour

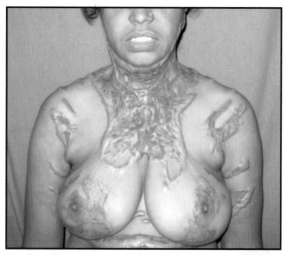

Fig. 14.23A: Hypertrophic scarring neck and chest

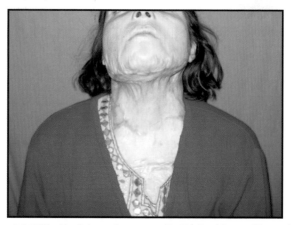

Fig. 14.23B: Excision of scars with thick skin grafting with well settled grafts

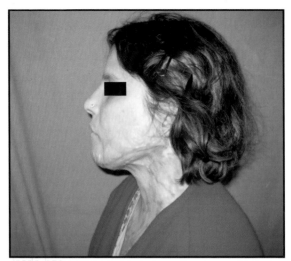

Fig. 14.23C: Lateral view of same patient

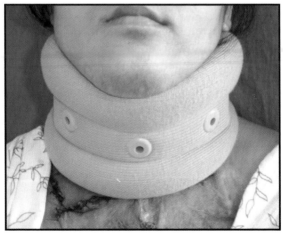

Fig. 14.23D: Soft collar to be worn at all times for at least 1 year to prevent secondary graft contracture

Breast

Breast contractures need to be released in girls of pubertal age group when there is just sufficient breast tissue so that further growth of the breast is not retarded. The incision should be in inframammary line and resurfacing is done with thick skin grafts. The graft is prevented from contracting by giving a conformer to the patient which maintains the position of the breast also (Figs 14.24A and B).

The nipple and areola if lost is to be reconstructed either by tattooing or sharing from the other normal breast or by grafting the areola by using labia majora graft. Nipple reconstruction is done using flaps from the same grafted skin or placing a silicone implant or dermafat graft under it. But nipple reconstruction is difficult in a completely grafted or scarred skin (Figs 14.25A to E).

Axilla, Elbow and Knee Contractures

- Released by Z- plasty or flaps.
- Simple release and grafting over the joints is difficult to maintain postoperatively by continuous use of splints (Figs 14.26A to C) because these are most mobile joints, therefore, if some local flap (Figs 14.27A to C) is given over the joint, chances of recontracture can be avoided and splint need not be worn for a long time postoperatively.
- Bi-pedicle releasing technique is also useful in straight joints. In this two incisions are given across scar contractures; parallel to each other, on either side of the joint with normal skin in between them. The

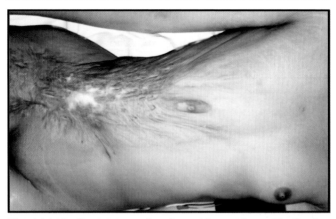

Fig. 14.24A: Contracture of groin and breast in continuity due to burns sustained in childhood. Breast development affected by the contracture

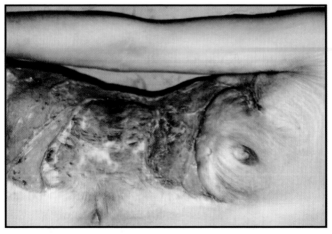

Fig. 14.24B: Release of contracture and split skin grafting bringing breast to its normal position

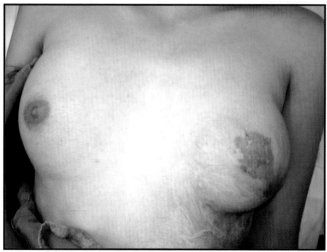

Fig. 14.25A: Post-burn scarring chest with loss of nipple and areola left side

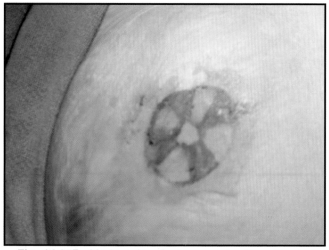

Fig. 14.25B: Marking for nipple reconstruction. Shaded areas to be de-epithelialized

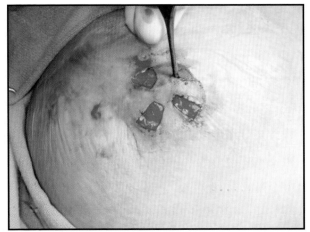

Fig. 14.25C: Alternate normal and de-epithelialized areas. The de-epithelialized areas are closed with sutures after pulling up the central island of skin and undermining the normal skin wedges

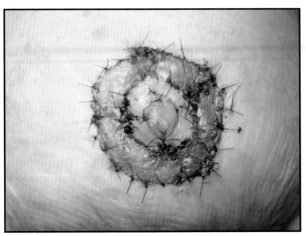

Fig. 14.25D: Immediate postoperative picture showing nipple and grafted areola.Graft for areola taken from labia majora

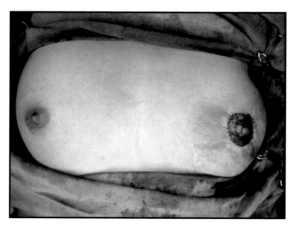

Fig. 14.25E: Two weeks postoperative
picture of same patient

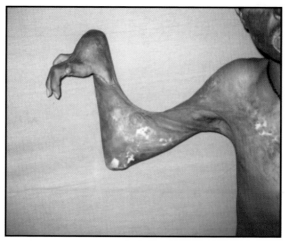

Fig. 14.26A: Typical deformity due to contracture of axilla, elbow
and hand in a young boy due to burns sustained in childhood

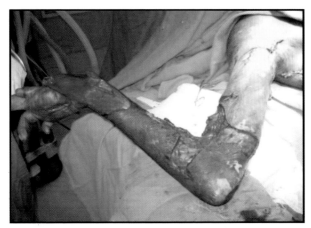

Fig. 14.26B: Release of wrist, elbow and axilla in single stage. However, complete release of elbow and wrist not possible due to tightening of muscles and tendons which can only be corrected by gradual splintage postoperatively

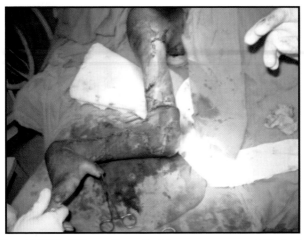

Fig. 14.26C: Skin graft applied to raw areas and Z-plasty in axillary contracture band

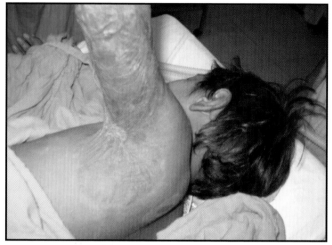

Fig. 14.27A: PBC axilla

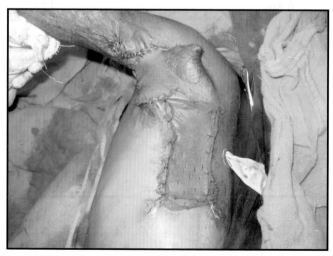

Fig. 14.27B: Released axilla and covered with
parascapular flap

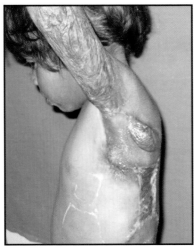

Fig. 14.27C: Three weeks postoperative picture with flap in place in axilla. Therefore postoperative splintage is not required

released areas are skin grafted. Therefore the chances of recontracture are less because the contracting grafts on either side of normal skin pulls the normal skin over the joint which thus acts as a flap (Figs 14.28A to 14.29B).

Hand

- Hand contractures need urgent attention if severe. In mild finger contractures on palmar side, either Z- plasty or release and skin grafting suffices followed by post-operative splintage.
- In mild to moderate dorsal contractures due to hypertrophic scarring of dorsal skin, excision of all scars and applying thick skin graft is sufficient (Figs 14.30A to 14.31B).

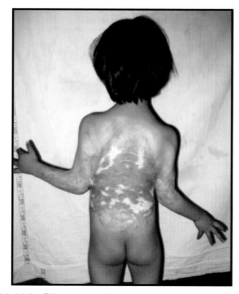

Fig. 14.28A: Bilateral axillary contractures, both anterior and posterior

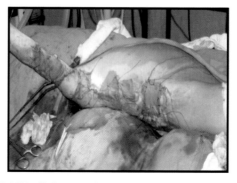

Fig. 14.28B: Release of contracture and grafting on raw areas created on arm, chest and interposed flap in axilla

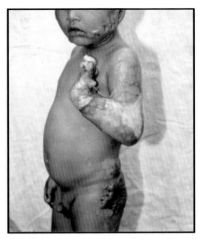

Fig. 14.29A: PBC elbow and hand in a 2 years old child

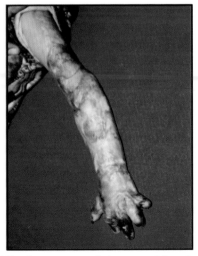

Fig. 14.29B: Contracture of dorsum of hand and elbow
released in first stage and grafted. Full function restored

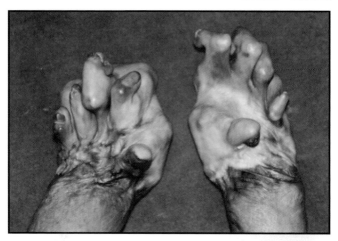

Fig. 14.30A: Typical PBC deformity both hands which are very difficult to correct

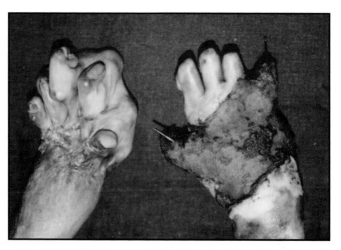

Fig. 14.30B: Release of dorsal contracture of one hand with skin grafting

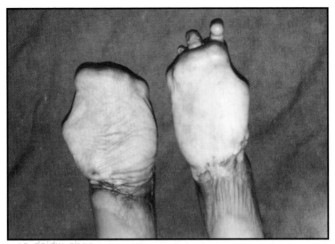

Fig. 14.30C: Volar aspect of both hands showing reversal of metacarpal arch

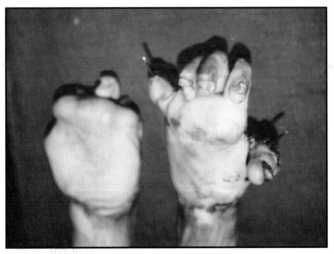

Fig. 14.30D: Arch reversal corrected in operated hand

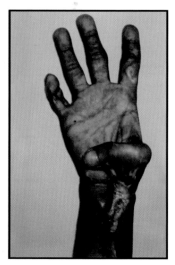

Fig. 14.31A: Adduction contracture
of thumb restricting use of hand

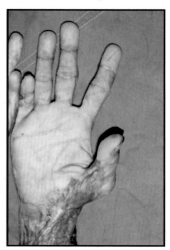

Fig. 14.31B: Release and grafted thumb

- In severe dorsal contractures where there is reversal of metacarpal arch, a simple release and skin graft is not sufficient because capsulotomies are required to mobilize MCP joints for which flap cover is essential over the dorsum of hand. Flaps used can be either posterior interosseous flap or groin or abdominal flap (Figs 14.32A and B).

- The second common deformity is web formation or syndactylization between fingers following burns. Web spaces can be released by multiple Z plasties or V - M plasty or five flap technique.

- In case of syndactylization of digits, flaps are created from dorsal side and raw surfaces on sides of fingers are covered with split skin graft.

- First web space contracture requires early attention because scar contracture in first web is associated with adductor muscle contracture. This can be corrected by release and split skin grafting or using a dorsal skin flap or a distant flap if the entire dorsum of the hand is scarred.

- The third common deformity in hand is the Boutonneir's deformity of fingers with loss of extension at proximal inter phalangeal (PIP) joints. Deep burns over the extensor aspect of finger causes the extensor hood over the PIP joint to become thin or absent so that the intrinsic muscles become flexors of PIP joints rather than extensors. As a result the lateral bands slip volarly which causes flexion at PIP joint and extension at DIP joint.

Early Boutonneir's deformity can be managed by simple splinting alone, which maintains PIP joint in

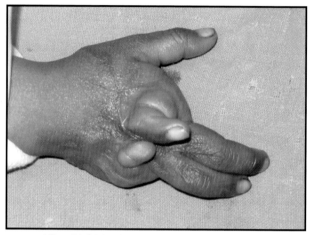

Fig. 14.32A: Dorsal contracture of fingers

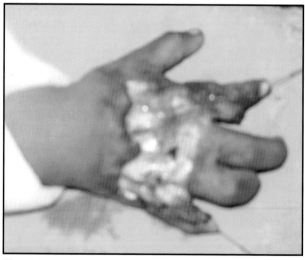

Fig. 14.32B: Released dorsal contracture with exposed
tendons requiring flap cover

extension allowing free movement of MCP joint. This splint is to be worn continuously for six weeks and then as night splint only till active extension is possible.

Chronic Boutonneir's deformity requires surgical correction through dorsal incisions if dorsal skin is normal or through midlateral incisions if dorsal skin is unstable. The extensor hood can be reconstructed by approximating the distal end of one lateral band which is volarly displaced, with proximal end of central band (Littler's I) or proximal end of one lateral band with distal end of central band (Littler's II).

Feet

Dorsal contractures of foot cause hyperextension of MTP joints which can be released and grafted. Rarely in severe contractures, the deep structures are also shortened which prevents complete correction of the contracture by the skin incision alone. This can be managed either by lengthening of tendons which requires a flap cover or post-grafting gradual traction and splintage can bring the foot to the correct position. Flap if required is usually raised from ipsilateral leg as a distally based fasciocutaneous flap or if the ipsilateral leg skin is also severely scarred, then contralateral leg is used to raise a cross leg flap.

CHAPTER 15

Firecracker Injuries

Firecracker injuries are seen in India commonly during Diwali and in the Western countries during New Year celebrations. Diwali, a festival of joy often becomes an occasion for sorrow and pain if proper safety precautions are ignored. The firecrackers can lead to a variety of injuries, if used indiscriminately and if lit improperly and carelessly.

Majority of the injuries are seen in >25 years age group but pediatric age group patients are also found in increasing numbers if they are not supervised by adults.In majority of the patients the injury is of emitting type - 'Anar' or 'flower pot', followed by exploding type - 'Bomb'. Apart from these injuries, there can be minor or major thermal burns by the clothes catching fire when lighting crackers.

The commonest means of lighting the crackers is by incense sticks and sparklers, followed by match sticks and candles and since these have significant ignition variation, the victims are often unsure of lighting firecrackers leading to sudden injuries, thus giving no time to retract themselves. In case of 'Anar', there is often a sudden bursting of the Anar on ignition which is a deviation from their normal emitting nature, therefore giving no time for safety.

Clinical Signs

The Anar burns usually involve the hands and face and are in the form of superficial to deep burns. The exploding 'Bombs' usually cause lacerated wounds in the hands. At times the damage is more severe if the bomb explodes in the hand itself. In such cases there is explosion of the tissues in the hand leading to multiple fractures of hand bones and even loss of skin and bones. Eyes are very often involved due to the bursting of the crackers and bombs leading to phosphorus burns (Figs 15.1 and 15.2). The self propelling Rockets are also known to cause severe damage if they are misdirected accidentally and can be responsible for major fires if they land up in any inflammable materials instead of going into the air and bursting in the sky.

Management

For superficial burns the management is the same as for any minor or major thermal burn depending on extent of burn surface. Since these burns are usually superficial, pain relief is very important.

For lacerations in hands (Figs 15.3 and 15.4), suturing is done to reposit the tissue back to as normal as possible.In case of major hand trauma, as much of bone and soft tissue as possible is to be saved. Fracture bones have to be fixed by K-wires or mini plates and exposed bones may require a flap cover.For this Groin flap is usually the workhorse flap. The others being abdominal flap or radial forearm flap or tensor fascia lata flap depending on the extent of damage.

Eyes have to be examined in case of facial burns for particulate materials used in the making of crackers. Phosphorus particles have to be removed manually and by saline irrigation and fluorescein staining done for corneal involvement.

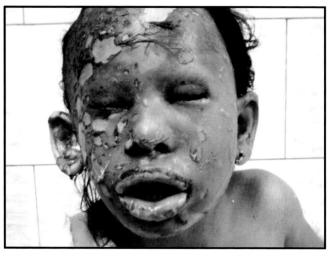

Fig. 15.1: Facial burns due to sudden bursting of "Anar"

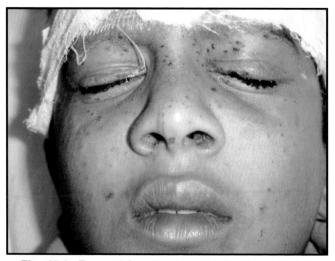

Fig. 15.2: Eye and face involvement due to particulate material present in the bombs

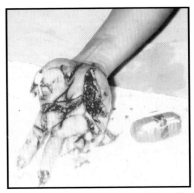

Fig. 15.3: Explosion of bomb in hand leading to multiple lacerations and fracture/amputation at various levels along. Also showing the bomb causing the injury

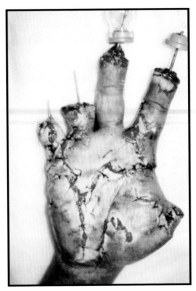

Fig. 15.4: Same hand as in Figure 15.3 after repair of lacerations and fixing fractures

Prevention of Firecracker Injuries

Though we cannot expect total elimination of firecracker injuries, the incidence and severity can definitely be reduced by keeping in mind the unpredictable nature of firecrackers especially 'Anar'. Also strict quality enforcing measures along with restrictive legislations regarding sale will reduce the incidence of these injuries. School campaigns can spread awareness amongst kids which will help in controlling use of firecrackers by children. Lastly, if firecrackers are lit in a common public ground by professionals for collective public enjoyment, it will not only reduce incidence of firecracker injuries but also go a long way in preventing unnecessary expenditure.

INDEX